ANATOM

WHAT T

Anatomical Terms and What They Mean

Professor TM Mayhew
University of Nottingham

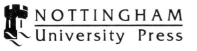
NOTTINGHAM
University Press

Nottingham University Press
Manor Farm, Main Street, Thrumpton
Nottingham, NG11 0AX, United Kingdom

NOTTINGHAM

First published 2001
© TM Mayhew

British Library Cataloguing in Publication Data
Anatomical Terms and What They Mean:
Mayhew, T.M.

ISBN 1-897676-79-4

Typeset by Nottingham University Press, Nottingham
Printed and bound by The Cromwell Press, Trowbridge, Wiltshire

PREFACE

My family name is Mayhew and is derived from the name Matthias which, in Hebrew, means 'gift of God'. This meaning may still hold appeal for my parents but I doubt whether any of my students see me in this light! The point is, although Mayhew has a meaning beyond merely identifying me as a member of this family line, that meaning has been lost over time. Occasionally, the meaning of a name has remained transparent. For example, we still recognise Smith as an occupational name even though its present owners may not pursue that occupation. In a sense, this book is about uncovering the mysteries of words and names.

An enterprise such as this may be justified in various ways. Basically, I enjoy words and their meanings and, for me, this has been justification enough. However, there is a more practical reason. Over the past 20 or so years in which I have taught Anatomy to medical and science students, it has become increasingly obvious that students are losing sight of the linguistic context in which anatomical terms and English words exist. In the case of students for whom English is the Mother tongue, the loss is explicable by the decline in teaching of Latin and Greek, languages whose influences on English and anatomical terminology are enormous. For overseas students in the UK (most of whom are from the Middle and Far East), the meaning and significance of anatomical terms may be even more opaque. Often, this is because they have less cultural exposure to Latin and Greek or even to the Romance languages (French, Italian, Spanish) which are, themselves, heavily influenced by Latin.

Here is a real example: I once examined a student from the Far East on the anatomy of the upper limb and, whilst she identified the structures which I pointed out, she was exceptionally slow in naming them. After a few minutes, I stopped the exam to enquire what the problem was. She responded that, having identified a structure, she next had to translate a mnemonic into the proper name. To understand her process, I asked her to talk me through how she identified (correctly) the **extensor carpi radialis longus** muscle. She recalled this name via the mnemonic **E**lephants **C**an **R**emember **L**atin and then had to decipher **E** for extensor, **C** for carpi and so on!

In other words, **extensor carpi radialis longus** had as much explanatory significance to her as elephants can remember Latin! We resumed the viva, giving her a little more time to answer each spotter question, and she passed comfortably.

To those who, like me, have had a minimal or amateurish exposure to Latin or Greek, much of anatomical terminology has a layer of meaning which is transparent from the words themselves. Thus, the student above would have found it much easier and quicker to link the structure and name if, on observing two extensor muscles (**extensor**) of the wrist (**carpi**) on the same side of the forearm as the radius (**radialis**), she noted that one (**longus**) was longer than the other. In similar fashion, the name **latissimus dorsi** muscle should tell the reader that this is a very extensive (**latissimus**) muscle of the back (**dorsi**). The term **cricoid** should tell the reader that this laryngeal cartilage is ring (**cric-**) shaped (**-oid**). Actually, it has the shape of a signet-ring, with an anterior band and a posterior plate. The name **azygos** vein should inform that this vein has no (**a-**) pair or partner (**-zygos**) on the right-hand side of the posterior thoracic wall.

Sometimes, anatomical terminology lets us down because of sloppy description, misspelling, abbreviation or the inevitable advances of time or technology. As an example of sloppy application, note that a cerebral **hemisphere** does <u>not</u> have the shape of a half-sphere; contrary to what its name suggests, the **innominate** bone of the pelvis - no (**in-**) name (**-nominate**) - <u>does</u> have a name! A widespread but disastrous misspelling is that of **fetus**: the incorrect **foetus** means 'something that stinks' but the correct **fetus** means 'something brought forth in pregnancy'. For an example of abbreviation, note that **skeleton** is short for **skeleton soma** which means 'the dry part of the body'. Finally, nowadays, it is not obvious why a **clavicle** was named because of its resemblance to a little key or why a **fibula** resembles a pin.

In an attempt to compensate for some of this obscurity, I have compiled a **glossary** (from Latin **glossa** 'word requiring explanation' and Greek **glossa** 'tongue', the same word-root which gives **hypoglossal** nerve, **glossopharyngeus** muscle, etc). The glossary is not exhaustive but embraces the most common and useful anatomical names, prefixes and suffixes. Emphasis is given to words which assist understanding. Therefore, words like artery (Latin for 'artery') and pharynx (Greek for 'pharynx') are excluded because they offer no added value. To examples of anatomical usage of a word-root, I have added other (often everyday) words of similar derivation just to emphasise that these "dead" languages are alive and well in modern English and in other areas of science. I very much hope that this compendium will allow students of Anatomy to make more sense of, and take more delight in, this fascinating and crucial activity. Note I said activity and not subject. Anatomy is something to be performed – it means cutting (**-tomy**) up (**ana-**)!

ABBREVIATIONS

Arab: Arabic
Gael: Gaelic
Gr: Greek
It: Italian
L: Latin
ML: Medieval Latin
OE: Old English
ON: Old Norse or Norwegian
Sp: Spanish

a: artery; aa: arteries
CNS: central nervous system
IVC: inferior vena cava
lig: ligament
m: muscle; mm: muscles
n: nerve; nn: nerves
SVC: superior vena cava
v: vein; vv: veins

REFERENCES

I have found the following reference texts extremely useful:

A New System of Anatomy. A Dissector's Guide and Atlas, Zuckerman S. Oxford University Press, Oxford, 1981

Collins Gem Latin Dictionary, Kidd DA. Collins, London & Glasgow, 1984

Collins Pocket Greek Dictionary, Watts N & George-Papageorgiou H. Harper-Collins, Glasgow, 1997

Engelsk Lommeordbok, Kunnskapforlaget, Oslo, 1999

Eureka!, Mary Byrne, Guild Publishing, London, 1987

Gray's Anatomy, 37th edition, ed Williams PL, Warwick R, Dyson M & Bannister LH. Churchill Livingstone, Edinburgh, 1989

The New Oxford Dictionary of English, ed Pearsall J. Oxford University Press, Oxford, 1998

Pocket Dictionary of the Latin & English Languages, MacFarlane P. Eyre & Spottiswoode, London, 1955

ACKNOWLEDGEMENTS

I dedicate this little book to all my students, past and present, at Nottingham University Medical School and elsewhere, who have encouraged me to learn more about the 'naming of parts' and 'meanings of words'. I am grateful to my Latin master at School, Mr JE Taylor (nickname 'Joe Soap' – but that's another mystery!). I thank my mentors, the late Prof Robert Barer (Sheffield) and Prof John Clegg (Aberdeen), who fostered my learning of Anatomy in their Departments. I thank my friends, Bob Banks (Durham), Reidar Myklebust (Tromsø), Albrecht Reith (Oslo) and Mick Turton (Sheffield), who share my love of words and/or stimulated my interest in Latin, Greek and Norwegian. Finally, I thank my parents (Doris, Leslie), my wife (Joan) and my family (Nick, Gemma, Zoë) for their love and sufferance.

GLOSSARY 1

SOME PREFIXES AND SUFFIXES
WORTH REMEMBERING

A-, An-: [Gr] prefix negating what follows. For example, someone who is not political is said to be apolitical. As an anatomical example, the azygos v (draining intercostal spaces on the right side of the posterior thoracic wall) has no equivalent structure on the left (azygos means 'having no pair or partner'). Intercostal spaces on the left drain instead into a set of hemiazygos vv.

Ab-: [L] denotes *from, away from, the opposite*. Something 'opposite to normal' is abnormal; someone who abstains will 'refrain from' doing something; to absorb is to 'suck [liquid] from'. In Anatomy, moving the upper limb away from the side of the body is abduction (abduction means 'drawing away from').

Ad-: [L] signifies *towards, near, next to*. Adjacent means 'lying close by'; ad infinitum means 'going towards infinity' or 'going on forever' (like one of my lectures!). In anatomical terms, moving the upper limb towards the side of the body is adduction (adduction means 'drawing towards'); the adrenal glands really are 'near the kidneys'.

Ana-: [Gr] prefix indicating *up*. To perform an anatomy ('cutting up') originally meant to perform a dissection; anabolism ('building up') is constructive metabolism in which complex molecules are synthesised from simpler precursors, e.g. anabolic steroids promote the build-up of muscle.

Ante-: [L] signifies *before* (in time, space or comparison), *in front*. An antenatal visit occurs 'before birth'; ante meridiem (am) means 'before midday'. In Anatomy, anterior means 'in or at the front'; the antebrachium is the 'forearm'; anteflexion of the uterus is 'forward flexion'.

Anti-, Ant-: [Gr] denotes *against, opposing, opposite*. Anticlockwise is 'opposite of clockwise'; an antiperspirant 'opposes sweating'; an antibody acts 'against a body [an antigen]'. In Anatomy, an antagonist ('fighter against') is a muscle with an opposite effect or action, e.g. triceps brachii m (elbow extensor) is an antagonist of biceps brachii m (elbow flexor).

Apo-: [Gr] means *from, away, by, off*. An apostle is a 'person sent away [to preach the gospel]'; an apothecary 'puts away or stores' drugs. An aponeurosis (literally, 'from muscle' or 'from tissue') is a flattened tendon arising from a muscle, e.g. the bicipital aponeurosis from biceps brachii m; during apocrine ('breaking off') secretion, pieces of cytoplasm are lost, e.g. secretion of milk by mammary gland cells.

Auto-: [Gr] meaning *self, own, same*. An automobile should be 'self-moving' (and not require a push or pull!); it may be an automatic 'acting of itself'; cell autolysis is 'self destruction'. The autonomic ('following its own laws') nervous system is involuntary, operating independently of the will.

Bi-, **Bis**-: [L] indicates *two, twice*. A bicycle has 'two wheels'; biscuit means 'twice-cooked' (originally this involved an initial bake followed by drying in a slow oven). The biceps brachii m has 'two heads'; the bicuspid valve has 'two points' like a mitre, the hat of a bishop (hence the alternative name, mitral valve!). Related to **Di**- (see below).

Circum-: [L] means *round, about*. Circumcision involves 'cutting around'; the circumference 'passes around' a circle; circumnavigators 'sail around' the World. In Anatomy, circumduction at the shoulder joint is a movement in which the limb is 'drawn around' in a circle with successive flexion, abduction, extension and adduction at the joint; circumflex means 'bending around', e.g. the circumflex branch of the left coronary a bends around the left border of the heart to pass posteriorly.

-**cle**, -**culus**, -**cula**, -**culum**: [L]: suffixes denoting *small, little*. A funicular ('using little ropes') railway runs up and down a slope using cables which counterbalance the carriages going up and down; cells have an endoplasmic reticulum ('little network') for protein synthesis and export. Similarly, in Anatomy, we have auricle ('little ear'), follicle ('small bag'), colliculus ('little hill'), retinacula ('little stays or ties' to bind down tendons) and trabecula ('little beam or strut').

Di-: [Gr] prefix indicating *two, twice*. A dioxide has 'two oxygen atoms'; dichromatic means having 'two colours'. In Anatomy, the digastricus m possesses 'two bellies'. Related to **Bi**-, **Bis**- (see above).

Dia-: [Gr] means *across, through, between*. The diameter of a circle or sphere is the 'right across measurement'; it is no coincidence that we say of a particular food "It went straight through me!" – diarrhoea means, literally, 'a flowing through'. The diaphragm ('fence between') separates the thorax from the abdomen; the diaphysis of a long bone is its shaft – diaphysis means 'between the growth regions'. See **epi**- below.

Endo-: [Gr] indicates *within*. An endoskeleton is inside the body; an endocrine ('secreting inwards') gland secretes into the bloodstream; the endoderm ('inner skin or layer') is the innermost germ layer; endocardium ('innermost heart [region]') really is the innermost layer of the heart.

Epi-: [Gr] denotes *on, near, upon, above, over, after*. Ephemeral means 'lasting only one day'; an epidemic ('on the people') affects many people in a given area. The epiphysis ('on the growth region') of a long bone lies on the growth plate and underlying growth region (metaphysis); epithelium (literally 'on the nipple') actually covers many other surfaces as well!

Exo-, **Ex**-: [Gr] means *external, outside, beyond*. The Exodus involved the Israelites finding a 'way out' of Egypt; exotic means 'out of the ordinary'; exogenous means 'having an outside origin'. Expiration is the 'breathing out' phase of mechanical respiration.

Hyper-: [Gr] means *above, over, in excess*. A hypercritical individual is 'overly critical'; a child who is "hyper" (short for hyperactive) is 'overactive'; a hypermarket is above an ordinary market (at least in size). Hyperplasia ('excessive creation') is cell division above the normal rate.

Hypo-: [Gr] signifies *below, beneath, down*. A hypocrite is 'not critical enough' (he/she doesn't include themselves!); formulating a hypothesis ('placing down') involves setting down an idea for testing. In Anatomy, the hypophysis (pituitary) arises as a 'downgrowth' from the hypothalamus ('below the thalamus'); in at least part of its course, the hypoglossal n is seen running 'below the tongue'.

-iform: [L] suffix indicating *of a certain shape or form*. Same as – **oid** [Gr] (see below). Falciform ('sickle-shaped') ligament; fusiform ('spindle-shaped'); piriform ('pear-shaped') recess; pisiform ('pea-shaped') bone.

Infra-, infero-: [L] prefix signifying *below, beneath, after*. Something infra dig is 'below one's dignity'; infrastructure is the 'underlying structure' of a system. The infraglenoid tubercle lies 'below the glenoid cavity'; the infraspinatus m lies 'below the spine [of the scapula]'; inferomedial means 'below and closer to the midline'.

Inter-: [L] indicates *between, among*. Intercourse is 'business between [individuals]' and may involve doing business or "doing the business"!; the interim is the 'between time'. The intertubercular groove of the humerus lies 'between the [greater and lesser] tubercles'; the interclavicular ligament runs 'between the clavicles'. Not to be confused with **intra**- (see below).

Intra-: [L] means *within, inside*. Something intramural lies 'within these walls'; intracellular means 'inside the cell'. Intraocular ('inside the eye') pressure increases in glaucoma. Not to be confused with **inter**- (see above).

Meso-: [Gr] indicates *middle, intermediate, between*. Mesopotamia was the land 'between the rivers' Tigris and Euphrates; in particle physics, a meson is a 'between particle' with a mass between an electron and a proton. The mesencephalon is the 'midbrain'; the mesoderm is the 'middle [germ] layer'. Note that meso- in Anatomy is also an abbreviation for mesentery, e.g. mesoappendix, mesocolon and mesosalpinx (mesenteries of appendix, colon and uterine tube respectively).

Meta-: [Gr] prefix with various meanings including *changing, transcending, going beyond*. Metabolism (the chemical 'change processes' of the body); metaphysics (something 'beyond physics'). The metaphysis of a bone is the 'growth change' region; the metacarpal bones are in the transition zone between the carpal (wrist) and phalangeal (finger) bones.

Mylo-: [Gr] signifies *associated with the molar teeth* (**mylos**: [Gr] molar). On the medial aspect of the mandible, the mylohyoid line runs downwards and forwards from posterior molars and provides attachment for the mylohyoid m. The mylohoid groove runs from the mandibular foramen to below the posterior molars and conveys the mylohyoid n to the muscle.

Myo-: [Gr] signifies *associated with muscle*. Myalgia ('muscle pain'), myology ('the study of muscle'), myocyte ('muscle cell'), myocardium ('muscle of the heart'), myosin (a muscle protein).

-oid: [Gr] suffix meaning *of a certain shape or form* (**eidos**: [Gr]). Cricoid ('ring-shaped') cartilage, mastoid ('breast-shaped') process, pterygoid ('wing-shaped') bone, scaphoid ('shaped like the keel of a boat') fossa of sphenoid ('wedge-shaped or wedged-in') bone; sesamoid ('seed-like') bones.

Para-: [Gr] prefix meaning *near, beside, passing alongside*. Parallel ('alongside one another') lines; paramedic (works 'alongside a medic'). In Anatomy, paranasal air sinuses are 'beside the nasal [cavity]' and open into it; the parasympathetic nervous system operates 'alongside the sympathetic system'; the parathyroid glands lie 'near the thyroid gland'.

Peri-: [Gr] indicates *around, surrounding, enclosing*. Perimeter ('the around measurement'); periscope (allows you to 'see around'). Pericardium invests the heart; the peritoneum is 'stretched around' the abdomen and its viscera; periosteum 'invests bone'.

Post-: [L] signifies *behind, after, following*. Postgraduation is a stage 'after graduation'; a postscript is 'written after' the main body of a letter. Posterior 'behind' is from this root.

Pro-: [Gr,L] means *before in time or position, forward*. To prostrate ('lay down in front of'); prothrombin (the 'precursor' of thrombin); to produce ('bring forward'). Amongst anatomical terms with this word-root are protraction ('drawing forwards') and protrusion ('thrusting forward').

Quadr-, Quadri-: [L] indicates *four*. A quadrangle has 'four angles' and a quadrat has 'four sides'. The quadratus femoris m is shaped 'like a quadrat' whilst the quadriceps femoris m has 'four heads'; the quadrangular space of the arm has 'four angles' and transmits the posterior circumflex humeral vessels and axillary n (of course, you remembered!).

Retro-: [L] indicates *back, backwards, behind*. Retroactive ('coming into effect from a date in the past'); retrogressive ('backward walking', i.e. going back to an earlier, and by implication, an inferior, state). Retraction ('drawing backwards') of the tongue is effected by styloglossus and hyoglossus mm. Retraction of the upper limb is brought about by the latissimus dorsi and other muscles.

Sub-: [L] denotes *under, beneath*. Sub-aqua sports involve going 'under water'; to subjugate is to 'put under the yoke'; subhuman is 'less than human'. The subarachnoid space lies 'below the arachnoid mater', between it and the pia mater; the sublingual gland lies 'beneath the tongue'; the subscapularis m is found 'under the scapula' when approached from posteriorly.

Super-, **supra-**: [L] means *above, over*. Superego (an 'above-normal ego'); supranational ('involving more than one nation'). Superior ('above') and suprarenal ('above the kidney') are anatomical terms from this same root.

Tri-: [Gr,L] indicates *three, three times*. A triangle has 'three angles'; a tripod has 'three legs'. The trigone is a 'triangular' area of bladder between the openings of the ureters and urethra.

Uro-: [Gr] signifies *associated with urine or the urinary system*. Urea (a product of protein metabolism excreted in urine), ureter (the tube conveying urine from the kidney to the bladder), diuretic (an agent stimulating flow of urine), urinal (a place or receptacle for passing urine), urology ('the study of the [genito-]urinary tract').

GLOSSARY 2

SOME USEFUL ANATOMICAL TERMS, MEANINGS AND USAGES

Anatomical Names	Latin/Greek or Other Origins	Examples
A.		
Abdomen, abdominal, abdominis	**Abdomen**: [L] *belly, paunch*; **abdominis**: [L] *of the abdomen*	Abdomen
		Transversus abdominis m
Abduction, abducent, abductor	**Abducere**: [L] *to lead away*	Abduction
		Abducent n (cranial VI)
		Abductor pollicis longus m
Acetabulum, acetabular	**Acetum**: [L] *vinegar*; **acetabulum**: [L] *vinegar cruet, cup-shaped vessel*	Acetabulum, acetabular fossa
		Acetabular labrum
Acinus, acini, acinar	**Acinus**: [L] *berry, grape, pip*	Serous and mucous acini
Acromion, acromial, acromio-	**Acros**: [Gr] *topmost, highest, outermost*; **omos**: [Gr] *shoulder*	Acromion

Anatomically, the abdomen is divisible into 9 regions: superiorly are the epigastric and left and right hypochondriac regions; intermediate are the umbilical and left and right lumbar (lateral) regions; inferiorly are the hypogastric and left and right inguinal (iliac) regions. What bony and other landmarks are used to define the horizontal and vertical lines between these regions?

Literally, the transverse muscle of the abdomen. It is the deepest of the 3 anterolateral muscles (what are the other two?) and is supplied by ventral rami of T7-T12 and L1 spinal nn. It helps to control intra-abdominal pressure. What are its attachments and how does a knowledge of these attachments help to explain why the muscle does not contribute to the layers of fascia covering the testis and spermatic cord?

To abduct a person is to kidnap him/her (take him/her away by force or cunning). Abduction of the upper limb moves it away from the midline of the body. Brought about by deltoid m and what other muscle?

The link here is that the abducent n supplies the lateral rectus m which abducts (laterally rotates) the eyeball.

The long abductor muscle of the thumb. Here, abduction is movement of the thumb to a position at which it is at right angles to the plane of the palm of the hand. What do you think the other thumb abductor m is called?

Acetic acid (the main ingredient of vinegar!). The acetabulum or acetabular fossa, is the deep pelvic cup which houses much of the head of the femur. Presumably, it resembles an ancient vinegar cup!

The fibrocartilaginous rim of the cup attached to the acetabulum and the transverse acetabular lig.

In parotid and pancreatic glands, the acini are arranged like bunches of grapes with the intercalated ducts being like the stalks.

Acrobat (walker on tip-toe), Acropolis (High City), acrostic (lines of poetry or other writing whose first letters spell out a word or phrase). The first letters of the cranial nn spell out O,O,O,T,T,A, F,V,G,V,A,H which gives a useful mnemonic: On Old Olympus's Towering Top…etc). The acromion is a bony lateral projection of the scapular spine which forms the 'tip of the shoulder'.

Anatomical Names	Latin/Greek or Other Origins	Examples
		Coracoacromial lig
		Acromioclavicular joint
Adduction, adductor	**Adducere**: [L] *to bring to, draw towards oneself*	Adduction
		Adductor brevis m
		Adductor pollicis m
Adenoid, adenoidal, adeno-	**Aden[as]**: [Gr] *gland*; **eidos**: [Gr] *shape, form*	Adenoids
		Adenohypophysis
Adipose, adipo-, adiposus	**Adeps**: [L] *fat*	Adipose tissue Adipocyte
		Panniculus adiposus
Aditus	**Aditus**: [L] *access, entrance, opening*	Aditus of the mastoid antrum
		Aditus of the larynx
Afferent	**Afferens**: [L] *carrying towards*	Afferent nerve
		Afferent lymphatic

The ligament between the coracoid process and acromion forming an arch over the shoulder joint.

A plane synovial joint between the lateral end of the clavicle and the medial side of the acromion. The joint houses an incomplete articular disc and is reinforced by acromioclavicular and coracoclavicular ligaments.

Adduce (to bring forth in evidence).

One of the adductors of the thigh at the hip joint. It is the smallest of the 3 muscles named adductor, the other 2 being? Adduction of the thigh involves moving it towards the midline.

An adductor of the thumb. This movement brings the thumb parallel to the side of the palm and to the fingers. Are there any other thumb adductors?

Adenoids (literally, gland-shaped), adenoidal (having swollen adenoids), adenoma (a tumour of glandular tissue). Anatomically, the term adenoids is confined to the lymphoid glands of the nose and nasopharynx (otherwise known as the pharyngeal tonsils).

Part of the hypophysis (pituitary gland). It comprises the pars anterior (or pars glandularis!), pars intermedia and pars tuberalis.

Adipose, adipocere (a waxy fat resulting from decomposition of the body under water), adipic acid (a fat derivative used in nylon manufacture). Adipose tissue is a connective tissue containing adipocytes (fat cells) specialized for fat storage. The two main types of adipose tissue are termed unilocular (white fat) and multilocular (brown fat). The 2 types differ in distribution and developmentally. How?

The fatty little web or network. Much white fat accumulates in the subcutaneous tissues or hypodermis where it is known as the panniculus adiposus. That of the abdomen may be several cm in thickness!

Adit (a term for an almost horizontal shaft into a mine). The aditus of the mastoid antrum connects the mastoid air cells to the tympanic (middle-ear) cavity.

Otherwise known as the laryngeal inlet. Its borders are antero-superior (the epiglottis), lateral (the aryepiglottic folds) and posteroinferior (the interarytenoid mucosal fold).

In Anatomy, afferent usually implies conveying neural information towards the CNS but is also used to describe blood or lymphatic vessels supplying an organ, gland or other structure, e.g. afferent lymphatics to lymph node, afferent arteriole to renal glomerulus.

Anatomical Names	Latin/Greek or Other Origins	Examples
Ala, alar	**Ala**: [L] *wing*	Alar ligaments
Alveolus, alveoli, alveolar	**Alveolus**: [L] *bath, basin, small sac, cavity*	Dental alveolus
		Alveolar nn
		Lung alveoli
Ampulla, ampullae	**Ampulla**: [L] *bottle, narrow-necked flask*	Ampulla of the uterine tube
Amygdala, amygdaloid	**Amygdalum**: [Gr,L] *almond*; **eidos**: [Gr] *shape*	Amygdaloid body
Anastomosis, anastomotic	**Ana-**: [Gr] *up, build up*; **stoma**: [Gr] *mouth*	Arterial anastomosis
Anconeus	**Ancon**: [L] *elbow*	Anconeus m
An[n]ulus, annular	**Anulus**: [L] *little ring*	Anulus fibrosus
		Annular ligament
Ansa	**Ansa**: [L] *loop, handle* (as on a jug)	Ansa cervicalis

Notes, Links and Non-Anatomical Usages

The 2 alar ligaments are strong ligaments which run like wings from the dens of the axis to the medial borders of the occipital condyles. They prevent excessive rotation at the atlantoaxial joints. Various other anatomical structures have a wing or ala, e.g. the cerebellum, crista galli of the ethmoid bone, sacrum, vomer.

The dental alveolus is the tooth socket.

These nerves supply teeth by entering their roots via their alveoli.

In section, the lung looks like a sponge – full of little spaces!

Ampullary. The ampulla of the uterine tube accounts for over half of total tube length and lies between the infundibulum and isthmus. It is thin-walled with a much-folded mucosa. Other structures also have ampullae, e.g. the vas deferens and semicircular canals.

Amygdalin (bitter-tasting extract from almonds). The amygdaloid body is in the walls of the inferior horn of the lateral ventricle in the temporal lobe of the cerebrum. It is associated with the sense of smell (olfaction) so should be particularly good at detecting cyanide which is found in bitter almonds!

Anastomosis (equipped with a mouth or junction), anastomotic. Anastomoses are circulatory safety devices to ensure continuity of flow to certain areas (e.g. arterial anastomoses) or devices for by-passing flow to certain regions (e.g. arteriovenous shunts).

Ancon (an architectural term for a bracket). The anconeus m (nerve supply?) is an extensor of the elbow.

Annulate. The an[n]ulus fibrosus (fibrous ring) is an important component of the intervertebral disc (the other being the nucleus pulposus which it encircles and contains). The anulus has outer collagenous and inner fibrocartilaginous zones. With advancing age, the anulus may weaken and the nucleus burst through, usually in a posterolateral direction. This happens in lumbago and sciatica.

The annular lig of the proximal radio-ulnar joint is a strong band which encircles the head of the radius keeping it against the radial notch of the ulna. Within the ligament, the radius is free to rotate. During which forearm movements does rotation occur?

The ansa cervicalis (loop of the neck) is formed by the union of an upper (spinal C1 and cranial XII nerves) and a lower (C2, C3 nerves) root which form a loop in front of the carotid sheath. It lies in which triangle of the neck?

Anatomical Names	Latin/Greek or Other Origins	Examples
Antagonist	**Ant-**: [Gr] *against;* **agon**: [Gr] *contest, struggle;* **agonistes**: [Gr] *rival, competitor*	Antagonistic muscle
Antrum, antral	**Antrum**: [L] *cave, cavern, hollow*	Pyloric antrum
		Mastoid antrum
Anus, anal, ani	**Anus**: [L] *ring, rectum*	Anus
		Anal sphincter
		Levator ani m
Aponeurosis	**Apo-**: *from, off;* **neuro**: [Gr] *nerve, muscle*	Palmar aponeurosis
Appendix, appendicular	**Appendix**: [L] *appendage*	Vermiform appendix
		Appendicular a

Notes, Links and Non-Anatomical Usages

Antagonism, antagonize, agony, agonist. Here, an antagonist is a muscle or muscle set which opposes the action(s) of another muscle or set. Antagonistic relationships may vary with the joint movement. Thus, in wrist flexion-extension, the flexors and extensors are antagonists but in adduction (medial or ulnar deviation) and abduction (lateral or radial deviation), some of the flexors are antagonists (e.g. flexor carpi ulnaris m versus flexor carpi radialis longus and brevis mm).

The pyloric antrum is caudal to the angular incisure of the stomach and leads into the pyloric canal which ends at the pylorus (opening into the duodenum).

An air sinus in the mastoid process of the temporal bone whose relations are surgically important because it can be infected. What are its anterior, posterior, superior, inferior, medial and lateral relations? It opens into the tympani cavity via the aditus of the antrum.

Not to be confused with anus: [L] old woman, or annus: [L] year (although the Queen's annus horribilis may have caused this senior citizen a pain in the backside!). Anulus (little ring) comes from this same word-root.

Has internal and external components. The internal sphincter is involuntary. The external is voluntary and has 3 parts: subcutaneous, superficial and deep. The internal sphincter is supplied by sympathetic nn from the inferior hypogastric plexus. What is the innervation of the external sphincter?

The main part of the pelvic diaphragm dividing the pelvis from the perineum. What is the other muscle of the diaphragm? The levator ani mm form a sling to support pelvic viscera and are supplied by the perineal branches of S4 and the pudendal n or the inferior rectal n.

An aponeurosis is a flat tendon arising from a muscle. In the case of the palmar aponeurosis, the muscle is palmaris longus which is absent on one or both sides in about 10% of people. Do you have a palmaris longus m? How would you find out?

Append, appendage. If the vermiform (worm-like) appendix is inflamed (appendicitis), it may need to be removed surgically (appendicectomy). But sometimes it is hidden from view! So what useful features of the colon might the surgeon follow to locate it?

Supplies the appendix as a branch of the posterior caecal a from the ileocolic a. What are the routes of venous and lymphatic drainage of the appendix?

Anatomical Names	Latin/Greek or Other Origins	Examples
Aqueous	**Aqua**: [L] *water*	Aqueous humour
Arachnoid	**Arachne**: [Gr] *spider, cobweb*; **eidos**: [Gr] *shape*	Arachnoid mater
Arcuate	**Arcus**: [L] *arch, bow, curve*; **arcuatus**: [L] *arched*	Arcuate ligaments
		Arcuate line
Areola, areolar	**Areola**: [L] *small open space*	Areolar tissue
		Areola of nipple
Articulation, articular	**Articulare**:[L] *to divide into joints, to speak distinctly*; **articulatio**: [L] *a joint*	Articulation
		Articular cartilage
Arytenoid, ary-	**Arytena**: [Gr] *funnel*; **eidos**: [Gr] *shape*	Arytenoid cartilages
		Aryepiglottic folds

Aqueous, aquatic, aqua vitae (water of life – a name given to intoxicating liquors in many languages, e.g. whisky derives from uisge-beatha [Gael] meaning water of life), aqueduct (water-channel – e.g. cerebral aqueduct). The aqueous humour fills the anterior and posterior chambers of the eye. It is produced by capillaries in the ciliary processs and drains away via anterior ciliary vv. Imbalances of production versus resorption may increase intraocular pressure. This condition is called what?

Arachnids (the class of animals that includes spiders and scorpions), arachnophobia (fear of spiders). The arachnoid mater is one of the 3 meninges covering the brain and spinal cord. Sandwiched between the outer dura mater and inner pia mater, it forms a delicate membrane deep to which is the subarachnoid space criss-crossed by a fine network of threads which resembles a spider's web!

The 5 curved arcuate ligaments (1 median, 2 medial, 2 lateral) attach the diaphragm to the posterior abdominal wall.

The arched line at which the anterior and posterior layers of the rectus sheath alter in composition, midway between umbilicus and pubic symphysis. Also, the iliac part of the linea terminalis which divides the greater from the lesser pelvis.

Areolar connective tissue is sometimes called loose connective tissue because of the open spaces seen on light microscopic examination.

The pigmented area of skin around the nipple which becomes larger and darker in females during pregnancy. Subareolar glands secrete a protective lubricant during lactation.

Article (a distinct item), articulate (able to speak well), articulation (synonymous with joint).

Found on the articular surfaces of bony elements in cartilaginous joints.

This is a mystery to me. The cartilages are not funnel-shaped but more like triangular pyramids. Perhaps the funnel, here, refers to the wide laryngeal opening (on the posterior summit of which the arytenoid cartilages sit) leading to the narrower tracheal lumen.

Mucosal folds running from the arytenoids to the epiglottis and containing muscle fibres (aryepiglottic mm, continuations laterally of the oblique arytenoid mm) and minor cartilages of the larynx.

Anatomical Names	Latin/Greek or Other Origins	Examples
Atlas, atlanto-	**Atlas**: [Gr] *a mythical Greek giant*	The atlas
		Atlanto-occipital joint
Atrium, atria, atrio-	**Atrium**: [L] *part of house next to entrance, hall* (i.e. where visitors are greeted)	Left and right atrium
		Atrioventricular valves
Audition, auditory	**Audire**: [L] *to hear*	Audition
		Auditory tube
		Auditory ossicles
Auricle, auricular[is], auriculo-	**Auris**: [L] *ear*, **auricula**: [L] *little ear, lobe of ear*	Auricle
		Auriculotemporal n
		Auricularis mm
Auscultation	**Auscultare**: [L] *to listen to*	Auscultation
Axilla, axillary	**Axilla**: [L] *arm-pit*	Axilla
		Axillary n

Notes, Links and Non-Anatomical Usages

The giant Atlas carried the World on his shoulders. The first cervical vertebra (the atlas) carries the head.

The joint between the superior articular facets of the atlas and the occipital condyles. The joint allows flexion-extension of the skull on the atlas with some lateral flexion. We nod our heads at atlanto-occipital joints but shake our heads at which other joints?

The atria are the receiving chambers of the heart!

Lie between atrium and ventricle. That on the left has 2 cusps and that on the right has 3. Coincidentally, the left lung has 2 lobes and the right has 3.

Audible, audience, audition (the special sense of hearing), auditorium, audio-cassette.

Joins the middle ear cavity to the nasopharynx, hence its alternative title - the pharyngotympanic tube.

Three tiny bones (ossicle means little bone) which run across the tympanic cavity from the tympanic membrane to the fenestra vestibuli. What are the names of the 3 bones?

Aural. The auricular appendages of the heart atria resemble little ears.

Sensory branch of the mandibular division of the trigeminal (cranial V) n supplying the skin of the ear and temple. Postganglionic (from which ganglion?) parasympathetic fibres of the glossopharyngeal (cranial IX) n hitch a ride on this nerve and leave it to provide secretomotor innervation to the parotid gland.

A set of very minor muscles which move the auricle of the ear and are supplied by the facial (cranial VII) n. They are often vestigial.

A form of examination involving listening to body sounds, usually with a stethoscope!

The axilla is a pyramidal region between the upper thoracic wall and arm. The anterior wall is formed by the pectoral mm, the posterior by subscapularis, teres major and latissimus dorsi mm and the medial by ribs 1-4 and their intercostal spaces and serratus anterior m. What structures form the lateral wall?

Provides the motor supply to the deltoid and teres minor mm. What is its cutaneous supply?

Anatomical Names	Latin/Greek or Other Origins	Examples
		Axillary tail
B.		
Biceps, bicipital	**Biceps**: [L] *two-headed*	Biceps brachii m
		Bicipital groove
Bicuspid	**Bicuspid**: [L] *having two points*	Bicuspid valve
Bifurcation	**Bifurcus**: [L] *two-forked*; **furca**: [L] *fork*	Bifurcation of the abdominal aorta
Brachium, brachial, brachio-	**Brachium**: [L] *arm*	Brachium
		Antebrachium
		Brachial a
		Brachialis m
		Brachioradialis m
Bregma	Uncertain. Maybe from **bregmenos**: [Gr] *wet, moist*	Bregma

Notes, Links and Non-Anatomical Usages

Runs from the superolateral quadrant of the breast along the lower border of pectoralis major m and towards the axilla and its pectoral group of lymph nodes.

Biceps brachii m (two-headed muscle of the arm) is a major flexor of the elbow joint and a powerful supinator when the elbow is flexed. Its long head runs in the intertubercular groove of the humerus and over the shoulder joint to the supraglenoid tubercle of the scapula. To which bit of the scapula does the short head attach?

Another name for the intertubercular groove.

The modern definition of bicuspid is having 2 cusps (rather than having 2 points). The bicuspid valve is the left atrioventricular or mitral valve.

Furcula (a forked structure such as the wishbone of a bird), bifurcate (divide into two forks or branches). The abdominal aorta bifurcates at the level of the 4th lumbar vertebra into the left and right common iliac aa.

Brachiate (swing from tree to tree using arms), Brachiosaurus (arm-lizard) was a dinosaur with forelimbs much longer than its hindlimbs. Anatomically, the arm extends from shoulder to elbow.

The forearm. It extends from elbow to wrist.

Arises from the axillary a as it enters the arm. It can be palpated medially as it lies on the brachialis m and is overlapped laterally by the biceps brachii m. To feel the pulse, push the latter muscle laterally and press laterally (not more deeply).

Arises from the anterio-inferior aspect of the humerus and inserts on the coronoid process of the ulna. It is supplied by the musculocutaneous n with 2 other muscles (why is it useful to remember BBC for the names of these 3 muscles?).

A flexor of the elbow and rotator of the forearm running from the lateral supracondylar ridge of the humerus to the lower lateral aspect of the radius. What is its nerve supply?

The area of the skull where the sagittal and coronal sutures meet. It may derive its name from the fact that this area feels soft and moist in the neonate because the frontal and parietal bones are unfused and surround the anterior fontanelle.

Anatomical Names	Latin/Greek or Other Origins	Examples
Brevis	**Brevis**: [L] *short, brief*	Adductor brevis m
Bucca, buccal, bucco-	**Bucca**: [L] *cheek, mouth*	Buccal n
		Buccopharyngeal fascia
Buccinator	**Buc[c]inator**: [L] *trumpeter*	Buccinator m
Bulla	**Bulla**: [L] *bubble, knob, stud*	Bulla ethmoidalis
Bursa	**Bursa**: [Gr, L] *skin, bag, pouch*	Subacromial bursa

C.

Caecum, caecal	**Caecus**: [L] *blind*	Caecum
Calcaneum, calcaneus, calcaneo-	**Calcaneum**: [L] *heel*	Calcaneum
		Tendo calcaneus
		Calcaneonavicular lig
Calvaria	**Calva**: [L] *skull*	Calvaria

Notes, Links and Non-Anatomical Usages

Brief, brevity. If a muscle is called X brevis, this implies that there is at least one other muscle called X longus. In the case of the femoral adductors, there is also a third, viz. adductor magnus m. Adductor brevis is the shortest of the 3 femoral adductor mm.

Buccal (concerning or related to the cheek). The buccal n is sensory to what areas of skin and mucosa?

The tough fascia covering the external surface of the pharynx.

Watch the cheeks of a trumpeter at full blow – the rounded cheek contours are contained by distended buccinator mm. What are the nerve supply and normal actions of this muscle?

Bull (as in 'papal bull' and from the same word-root as bulletin), bullet. The ethmoidal bulla is a promontory on the lateral wall of the nasal cavity (middle meatus) caused by the middle ethmoidal air sinuses.

Bursitis, bursar (treasurer of a college or university – holding on to the sack of money?), bursary (scholarship award – usually not a sack of money!). I have suffered from inflammation of the subacromial bursa (subacromial bursitis). Where do you think the bursa lies? Is it connected to the shoulder joint cavity? What are the effects of its bursitis?

Caecum (short for 'intestinum caecum' or blind ending of the intestine). Indeed, it is a cul-de-sac from which the appendix opens.

Calcaneum – the heel bone.

The tendo calcaneus (calcaneal or Achilles tendon) is the powerful tendon into which the gastrocnemius and soleus mm run. It inserts on the posterior aspect of the calcaneum.

The plantar calcaneonavicular (or spring) lig is very strong and rather elastic. It runs from the anterior of the sustentaculum tali of the calcaneum to the inferior of the navicular tuberosity and is the plantar ligament of the talocalcaneonavicular joint. It helps to maintain the medial longitudinal arch of the foot.

Calvary (the hill where Jesus Christ was crucified) comes from the same word-root since it is a translation, via Greek (Golgotha: [Gr] place of skulls), of the Aramaic word Gulgulta The term calvaria is now restricted to describe the skull cap. Calvities is a term used to describe baldness affecting the top of the head. Interestingly, calva [Sp] means bald!

Anatomical Names	Latin/Greek or Other Origins	Examples
Calyx, calyces	**Kalyx**: [Gr] *cup, case of a bud*	Renal calyx
Capitulum	**Capitulum**: [L] *small head*	Capitulum
Caput, capitis, capitate	**Caput**: [L] *head*	Caput Medusae
		Splenius capitis m
		Capitate bone
Cardiac	**Cardia**: [Gr] *heart*; **cardiacus**: [L] *relating to heart, or to upper part of stomach where the oesophagus enters*	Cardiac vv
		Cardiac notch of the lung
Carina	**Carina**: [L] *keel, ship*	Carina tracheae
Carotid	**Karotis**: [Gr] *drowsiness*	Carotid a
		Carotid bifurcation

Notes, Links and Non-Anatomical Usages

The minor calyces of the kidney are cup-like extensions of the pelvis into which the papillary ducts of nephrons open. Minor calyces unite to form major calyces which converge on the renal pelvis proper. From this, the ureter arises.

Capitulate (to draw up terms of surrender under various headings). The rounded capitulum at the distal end of the humerus articulates with the shallow fossa of the head of the radius.

Capital (main city), capitation (a poll tax or tax per head), captain (head person on board ship), decapitation ("Off with his head!"). One of the visible signs of portal hypertension is a set of swollen veins radiating from the umbilicus like the 'head of the Medusa' (caput Medusae), a mythical creature who had hissing snakes instead of hair!

An extensor and rotator of the head running from the mastoid process and superior nuchal line to the ligamentum nuchae and spinous processes of vertebrae C7-T3. It is supplied by dorsal rami of middle cervical spinal nn. It gets its name (bandage of the head) from its long, thin, strip-like appearance.

The capitate is the largest and, therefore, the head carpal bone.

Cardiology. The term cardia is used to refer to the oesophageal opening of the stomach. Cardiac vv drain the heart and (except for which veins?) mostly open into the right atrium via the coronary sinus.

Owing to the leftward disposition of the heart and pericardium, the anterior border of the left lung deviates to the left below the 4th costal cartilage and then curves down towards the 6th.

Carinate (having a keel). The carina of the trachea is the keel-like inferior part of the last (lowest) tracheal cartilage and runs in the gap created by the tracheal bifurcation into main bronchi. The term is sometimes used to refer to the bifurcation itself (vertebral level T4-T5).

The arteries were so-named from the belief that their compression caused drowsiness or stupor. The left common carotid a arises from the aortic arch. The right common carotid a arises where?

At the level of the upper border of the thyroid cartilage (corresponding to a horizontal plane passing through the disc between C3 and C4 vertebrae), the common carotid aa bifurcate into the internal and external carotid aa. The cervical part of the internal carotid a has no branches. But what are the branches of the external carotid a?

Anatomical Names	Latin/Greek or Other Origins	Examples
Carpus, carpal, carpi, carpo-	**Karpos**: [Gr] *wrist*; **carpere**: [L] *pluck, seize*	Carpal bones
		Flexor carpi ulnaris m
		Carpometacarpal joints
Caruncle	**Caruncula**: [L] *a small morsel of meat* (hence, *a small fleshy eminence*)	Lacrimal caruncle
Cauda, caudal, caudate	**Cauda**: [L] *tail*	Cauda equina
		Caudate lobe
		Caudate nucleus
Cavernous	**Caverna**: [L] *cave, hollow, cavern*	Cavernous sinus
Cephalon, cephalic	**Cephalon**: [Gr] *head*	Encephalon
		Mesencephalon
		Cephalic v

Carpe diem (seize the day! – to grip something tightly, you need to extend at the wrist). Carpus is the anatomical name for the wrist. What are the names of the carpal bones?

Flexor of the wrist on the ulnar (medial) side. Supplied by ulnar n.

Except for the first (that of the thumb), these are plane synovial joints allowing flexion, extension, adduction, abduction and some rotation. The joint of the thumb is a synovial saddle joint and also allows circumduction.

Caruncle (the fleshy outgrowth which is the cock's comb). The lacrimal caruncle is a reddish fleshy mass of skin at the medial angle of the eye and contains sebaceous and sweat glands.

Caudal implies closer to the tail. The cauda equina (horse's tail) arises because the spinal cord terminates in the upper lumbar region but lower spinal n roots have to travel progressively longer distances to their vertebral exits. The appearance in the vertebral canal is of a horse's tail!

A small lobe at the posterior of the visceral surface of the liver and sandwiched between the IVC and lesser omentum.

Together with the lentiform (lens-shaped) nucleus, it forms the corpus striatum (striated body) of the forebrain. The caudate (tail-bearing) nucleus has a head, body and tail.

Cave, cavern (a large cave). A cavernous venous sinus lies on each side of the body of the sphenoid bone and extends from the apex of the petrous part of the temporal bone to the superior orbital fissure. The nerves associated with its lateral wall are "O, Tom!" being, from above downwards, the Oculomotor (cranial III), Trochlear (IV), Ophthalmic (V) and Maxillary (V) nn. What other important structures are found associated with the sinus?

Cephalopod (foot-headed creature, like an octopus or squid, in which the feet or tentacles look as if they grow out of the head), Bucephalus (Oxhead – the favourite horse of Alexander the Great had a white, ox-like patch on its head), encephalogram (an image of the brain), hydrocephalus (water on the brain – cured by a tap on the head?). The brain (encephalon) is contained in the head.

The midbrain connects the pons and cerebellum (hindbrain or rhombencephalic structures) with the forebrain (prosencephalon).

Drains at the head-end of the arm rather than the bottom-end (basilic v). Into which vein does the cephalic v drain?

Glossary 2   **31**

Anatomical Names	Latin/Greek or Other Origins	Examples
Cerebellum, cerebellar	**Cerebellum**: [L] *small brain*	Cerebellum
		Cerebellar peduncles
		Tentorium cerebelli
Cerebrum, cerebral, cerebro-	**Cerebrum**: [L] *brain*	Cerebrum
		Cerebral cortex
Cervix, cervical[is]	**Cervix**: [L] *neck*	Uterine cervix
		Cervical vertebra
Chiasma, chiasmata	**Chiasma**: [Gr] *crossing-over*	Optic chiasma
Choana, choanae	**Choane**: [Gr] *funnel*	Choana
Chondral, chondro-	**Chondros**: [Gr] *cartilage, gristle*	Costochondral joint
Chorda, chordae	**Chorda**: [L] *cord, rope*	Chondrocranium
		Chorda tympani

Cervelat and saveloy sausages both come from this root and, presumably, once contained brain!

Stalks of projection fibres connecting the cerebellum to the midbrain (superior cerebellar peduncles), pons (middle) and medulla oblongata (inferior cerebellar peduncles) and, hence, to other sites.

The tent of the cerebellum is made of dura mater and covers the cerebellum in the posterior cranial fossa. It is attached to the occipital (posteriorly), temporal (laterally) and sphenoid (anteriorly) bones.

Cerebration (using the brain), decerebrate (having no brain, usually because it has been removed!).

Complexly folded into gyri and sulci. Although its surface is very extensive, about 2/3 of the total surface is hidden from view within the sulci and the insula.

The uterine cervix projects as a knob into the vagina and is surrounded by the fornix which is subdivided into anterior, posterior and lateral fornices. What pelvic structures can be palpated by inserting a finger into these fornices?

How many cervical vertebrae are there? How many does a giraffe have?

Ultimately stemming from resemblance to the Greek letter chi which is cross-shaped. Exactly the shape of the optic chiasma at which fibres from the nasal (medial) halves of the retina become contralateral whereas those from the temporal (lateral) halves remain ipsilateral. During meiosis, maternal and paternal chromatids swap genetic material in the process called chiasma formation or crossing-over!

The nasal choanae (posterior nasal apertures) funnel inspired air into the nasopharynx.

Chondrocyte, chondroblast, achondroplasia, chondrichthyes (the cartilaginous fish, including the sharks and rays). Costochondral joints occur between ribs and their cartilages. There is no movement between them since the cartilage is merely the unossified remnant of rib development from cartilage.

Parts of the skull developing or remaining in a cartilaginous state.

The chorda tympani (cord of the eardrum) is a branch of the facial n (cranial VII) which leaves the skull at the petrotympanic fissure and joins the lingual n. In part of its course, it runs across the medial side of the tympanic membrane.

Anatomical Names	Latin/Greek or Other Origins	Examples
		Chordae tendineae
Choroid	**Chorion**: [Gr] chorion; **eidos**: [Gr] form	Choroid (eyeball), choroid plexus (ventricles)
Ciliary	**Cilium**: [L] eye, eyelash; **supercilium**: [L] eyebrow	Ciliary body, ganglion, etc
Cingulate	**Cingula**: [L] belt, girdle	Cingulate gyrus
Cisterna	**Cisterna**: [L] reservoir, cistern	Cisterna magna
		Cisterna chyli
Clavicle, clavicular, clavi-, -clavian, -clavius	**Clavis**: [L] key, bolt, bar	Clavicle
		Clavipectoral fascia
		Subclavian aa
		Subclavius m
Cleido-	**Cleido-**: [Gr] relating to the clavicle	Sternocleidomastoid m

Tendinous cords passing from a given papillary mm to adjacent sides of an adjacent pair of cusps of an atrioventricular valve.

Choroid, at whatever site, resembles chorion in containing many blood vessels!

Cilia resemble tiny eyelashes, a supercilious person looks at you with raised eyebrows (and looks down the nose!). The ciliary body, ganglion and muscles are all associated with the eye.

Surcingle (a strap running round a horse to keep a rug in place), cinch (a girth for a Western saddle) comes from the same word-root via cincha: [Sp] girth. The cingulate gyrus lies on the medial aspect of the cerebrum and, with the cingulate sulcus, partly encircles the corpus callosum.

Cistern. The cisterna magna (big cisterna), otherwise known as the cerebello-medullary cistern, is a subarachnoid space containing cerebrospinal fluid.

This 'juicy cistern' is a narrow lymphatic (lymph is the juice) sac running posterior to the abdominal aorta and IVC and becoming continuous with the thoracic duct. Intestinal and lumbar lymphatic trunks from the intestines, lower limbs and lower trunk drain into it.

The collar-bone is the clavicle (little key – named because its shape resembles that of a key used by the ancients), clavichord (a keyboard instrument).

Deep fascia ensheathing the pectoralis minor and subclavius mm and attached to the clavicle and axillary fascia.

These arteries pass 'below the clavicle' and become the axillary aa as they pass into the axilla. The branches of the subclavian a are the vertebral a, thyrocervical trunk, costocervical trunk and internal thoracic a. What areas do they supply?

A small muscle running from the 1st rib and costal cartilage to the inferior surface of the middle third of the clavicle. The muscle is supplied by spinal nn C5 and C6 but an important function for the muscle is hard to find. It presumably depresses the lateral end of the clavicle.

This muscle attaches to the mastoid process and the sternum and clavicle. It is supplied by the accessory n. How would you test the muscle's action in a patient?

Anatomical Names	Latin/Greek or Other Origins	Examples
Coccyx, coccygeal	**Coccyx**: [L] *cuckoo*	Coccyx
		Anococcygeal body
		Coccygeus m
Cochlea, cochlear	**Cochlea**: [L] *snail, snail shell*	Cochlea
		Vestibulocochlear n (cranial VIII)
Coeliac	**Coeliacus**: [L] *related to the stomach*; **Koilia**: [Gr] *stomach, belly, abdomen*	Coeliac plexus
Coelom, coelomic	**Koilos**: [Gr] *hollow*; **koiloma**: [Gr] *cavity*	Coelom (or coelomic cavity)
Collateral	**Col-**: [L] *together with*; **latus**: [L] *side*	Fibular collateral lig
		Collateral circulation
Colliculus, colliculi	**Colliculus**: [L] *little hill*	Superior colliculus
Colon, colic, colo-	**Colon**: [L] *large intestine*	Colon

Notes, Links and Non-Anatomical Usages

In sagittal section, the coccyx is shaped like a cuckoo's beak.

A midline raphe for part of the levator ani m and lying between the coccyx and anus.

The posterolateral component of the pelvic diaphragm attached to the ischial spine and sacrococcyx and supplied by spinal nn S4 and S5.

The cochlea of the inner ear resembles a snail shell.

This nerve is associated with hearing (audition) and balance (equilibration). What artery accompanies the nerve into the internal acoustic meatus?

The coeliac plexus is the largest autonomic plexus found posterior to the stomach and surrounding the roots of the coeliac and superior mesenteric aa. Coeliac disease (a gluten hypersensitivity affecting the small intestine rather than the stomach).

The mesodermal body cavity containing abdominal and other viscera. The coelacanth (hollow spine) is a fish, once thought extinct, which has fins bearing hollow spines.

Collateral here has the sense of supportive. The fibular collateral lig is found on the fibular (lateral) side of the knee joint. Is this ligament attached to the lateral meniscus?

When the blood supply to a particular region is interrupted, compensatory circulations may open up. For instance, superior and inferior ulnar collateral aa arise from the brachial a and anastomose around the elbow joint with ulnar recurrent aa from the ulna a. The clinical importance of these collaterals becomes apparent when the brachial or ulna aa are obstructed near the elbow.

The superior and inferior colliculi together make up the corpora quadrigemina (the quadruplet bodies) and sit on the tectum of the midbrain.

Colonic irrigation (more a fashion statement than a therapy), colostomy (a surgical intervention to create an artificial opening from the colon to serve as an anus). The colon is distinguishable by the presence of taeniae coli, haustrations and appendices epiploicae!

Anatomical Names	Latin/Greek or Other Origins	Examples
		Colic aa
Commissure, commissural	**Commissura**: [L] *joint, connection*	Anterior commissure
		Commissural fibres
Condyle, condylar	**Kondylos**: [Gr] *knuckle*	Occipital condyle
		Bicondylar joints
Contralateral	**Contra**-: [L] *opposite*; **latus**: [L] *side*	Contralateral limb
Coracoid, coraco-	**Korax**: [Gr] *raven*; **eidos**: [Gr] *shape, form*	Coracoid process
		Coracobrachialis m
Cornu, cornua	**Cornu**: [L] *horn, hoof, beak, claw*	Cornua (of hyoid, thyroid, ventricles of brain)
Coronary, coronoid, coronal	**Corona**: [L] *crown, garland*	Coronary aa
		Coronoid process

Ascending colon is supplied by right colic aa from the superior mesenteric a; the middle colon is supplied by middle colic aa from the same source. But what is the source of left colic aa which supply the descending colon?

Commissar (an official enjoined or entrusted with a particular responsibility). The anterior commisure is a narrow but distinct bundle of commissural fibres running anterior to the columns of the fornix and below the lentiform nucleus. Its fibres fan out into the anterior part of the temporal lobe, including the parahippocampal gyrus.

Whilst all nerve fibres connect nerve cells to target tissues, not all are commissural in the strict sense since some are projection and others association fibres. Commissural implies connecting similar areas of left and right sides; projection implies connecting different CNS areas and association implies connecting different areas on the same side.

A condyle is a convex prominence at the end of a bone. The knuckles are formed by the bones of the metacarpo- and inter-phalangeal joints and their convex articular surfaces. The occipital condyles articulate with the atlas at the atlanto-occipital joints. What movements occur at these joints?

These have movement mainly in one plane but with limited rotation in a plane at right angles to the first.

On the opposite side of the body to the other limb.

An anterolateral projection from the scapula named for its resemblance to the beak of a raven.

Attaches to the coracoid process and medial humeral shaft.

The root implies anything horn-like. Several words come from this root including cornucopia (the mythical horn of plenty), cornea (the anterior covering of the eyeball), corniculate (minor cartilages of the larynx). The hyoid and thyroid cartilages have multiple horns (cornua).

Coronation (a crowning ceremony), coronet. The coronary aa pass around the heart like a crown. The left and right coronary aa arise where? Do they anastomose?

There are 2 such processes: one crowns the ramus of the mandible and provides attachment for the temporalis m; the other crowns the trochlear notch on the proximal end of the ulna.

Anatomical Names	Latin/Greek or Other Origins	Examples
		Coronal suture
Corpus, corpora	**Corpus**: [L] *body, flesh, corpse, substance*	Corpora quadrigemina
		Corpus callosum
		Corpus luteum
Cortex, cortical	**Cortex**: [L] *rind, shell, crust, bark, cork*	Cerebral cortex Adrenal cortex
Costal, costo-	**Costa**: [L] *rib*	Costal cartilage
		Costoclavicular lig
Cranium, cranial, cranio-	**Cranium**: [L] *skull*	Cranium
		Cranial nn (I to XII)
Cremaster	**Kremastos**: [Gr] suspended, hanging	Cremaster m
Cribriform	**Cribriform**: [L] *like a sieve or colander*	Cribriform plate
		Cribriform fascia of the thigh

Notes, Links and Non-Anatomical Usages

Coronal planes relate to the crown of the head and divide the body vertically into anterior and posterior parts, i.e. parallel to the coronal suture of the skull which separates the frontal and parietal bones (see frontal below).

Corporation, corps, corpse, corpulent, corpuscle. The 4 bodies which make up the corpora quadrigemina are the 2 superior and 2 inferior colliculi. Where are they found?

The corpus callosum (tough body) is a large mass of commissural tissue joining the 2 cerebral hemispheres.

Corpus luteum (yellow body) as opposed to corpus albicans (white body). Both bodies are found in which organ?

Cerebral cortex covers the cerebrum.
Covers the adrenal gland and produces corticosteroids.

Costard (a British variety of cooking apple which is large and ribbed). Costal cartilages of ribs 1-7 articulate with the sternum. With what do the cartilages of the other ribs articulate?

Runs from the inferomedial surface of the clavicle to the superior surface of the first rib and its costal cartilage. The ligament is an accessory ligament of the sternoclavicular joint.

Craniates (skulled animals), craniotomy (cutting into the skull).

Cranial nn: what do O,O,O,T,T,A,F,V,G,V,A and H stand for?

The muscle raises the testis and scrotum for protection and temperature regulation and so, in a sense, suspends the testis. The nerve supply is the genitofemoral n which also supplies skin on the medial aspect of the thigh. Stroking this skin elicits the cremasteric reflex – the contralateral testis rises. A really neat party trick! Butterfly pupae have a hook-shaped structure for purposes of suspension. Guess what, it's called the cremaster!

The cribriform plate of the ethmoid bone is pierced by many little holes which transmit nerve fibres from the nasal olfactory mucosa to the olfactory bulb.

Femoral superficial fascia over the saphenous opening is pierced by the great saphenous v and other vessels. This area is called the cribriform fascia.

Anatomical Names	Latin/Greek or Other Origins	Examples
Cricoid, crico-	**Krikos**: [Gr] *ring*; **eidos**: [Gr] *shape*	Cricoid cartilage
		Cricoarytenoid mm
Crista	**Crista**: [L] *a plume on crest of a helmet, crest, cock's comb*	Crista galli
		Crista terminalis
Crus, crura, crural	**Crus**: [L] *leg, shin*	Crus cerebri
		Crus of the diaphragm
Crux, cruciate, cruciform	**Crux**: [L] *cross*	Posterior cruciate lig
		Cruciform lig
Cubital	**Cubitum**: [L] elbow	Cubital fossa
		Median cubital v
Cuboid, cuboidal	**Kubos**: [Gr] *cube*; **eidos**: [Gr] *shape*	Cuboid bone

The cricoid cartilage is like a signet ring.

Laterals adduct, posteriors abduct the vocal cords. Of course, you remember their nerve supply!

Crest, crestfallen. The crista galli (literally, the cock's comb) is a superior projection from the ethmoid bone in the anterior cranial fossa to which the falx cerebri attaches.

Means boundary crest. It is the ridge on the interior of the right atrium running from the superior to the IVC opening. On one side of the ridge, the atrial wall is smooth; on the other, it is rough. The latter is due to muscular ridges (musculi pectinati) running anteriorly and into the auricular appendage.

The leg of the cerebrum on each side forms the anterior part of a cerebral peduncle. The crura convey corticospinal projection fibres that descend through the pons and into the medulla oblongata.

The leg of the diaphragm on each side attaches the diaphragm to the posterior abdominal wall. The left crus arises from L1 and L2 vertebrae. The longer right crus extends lower down (L1-L3 vertebra) and forms a sling around the lower oesophagus. The 2 crura unite to form a median arcuate lig behind which is the aortic hiatus (level T12, L1).

Crucial, crucifix, crucify, crusade (the crusaders wore tunics emblazoned with the holy cross). The anterior and posterior cruciate ligaments of the knee joint appear X-shaped when viewed from the medial or lateral sides. The ligaments stabilise the joint antero-posteriorly.

This has transverse and longitudinal components which hold the dens of the axis next to the anterior arch of the atlas (transverse element) and attach the atlas to the occipital bone and axis (longitudinal element).

Cubit (old measure based on forearm length). The boundaries of the fossa are the pronator teres m (medial) and brachioradialis m (lateral). In the middle is the tendon of biceps brachii m with the brachial a on its medial side.

This subcutaneous vein is so constant that it is a standard site for intravenous injection. It connects the basilic and cephalic vv of the upper limb.

Cubic, Cubism (an art form pioneered by Picasso and which made use of simple geometric shapes rather than perspective). The cuboid tarsal bone is rather cuboidal in shape.

Anatomical Names	Latin/Greek or Other Origins	Examples
Cuneus, cuneate, cuneiform	**Cuneus**: [L] *wedge*	Cuneiform bones
		Cuneus
		Cuneate fasciculus and cuneate tubercle
Cusp	**Cuspis**: [L] *point, spear, javelin*	Bicuspid valve
		Tricuspid valve
Cyst, cystic	**Kuste**: [Gr] *cyst, bladder*	Cystic duct

D.

Anatomical Names	Latin/Greek or Other Origins	Examples
Decussation	**Decussis**: [L] *the number 10 in Latin is X (decem);* **decussare**: [L] *to divide cross-wise*	Pyramidal decussation
Deferens	**Defero**: [L] *carrying to a place, bringing down/from*	Vas deferens
Deltoid	**Delta**: [Gr] *the Greek letter* Δ; **eidos**: [Gr] *shape*	Deltoid muscle, ligament
Dens, dental, dentate	**Dens**: [L] *tooth or anything of similar shape*	Dens
		Dentate gyrus

Notes, Links and Non-Anatomical Usages

Cuneiform (old form of writing using wedge-shaped symbols). When the distal articular surfaces of the 3 cuneiform bones of the tarsus are viewed, they look wedge-shaped. These bones, and their shape, contribute to the transverse arch of the foot.

This is a wedge-shaped region on the posteromedial aspect of the occipital lobe of the cerebral hemisphere. It lies between the calcarine and parieto-occipital sulci.

The cuneate tubercle is a lateral swelling at the rostral end of the cuneate fasciculus on the posterior of the medulla oblongata. The cuneate fasciculus is an ascending spinal tract and, on transverse section, it looks wedge-shaped.

The bicuspid (2 cusps) is the left atrioventricular valve.

This is the right atrioventricular valve and has 3 cusps.

Cyst, cystitis (bladder inflammation), cholecystitis (gall-bladder inflammation), cystoscope (for viewing the bladder). The cystic duct joins the gall bladder to the common hepatic duct to form the bile duct. The cystic duct has a mucous coat arranged as a spiral fold.

December (the tenth month in the Roman calendar!), decimal, decimate (to reduce by a factor of 10). The pyramids are promontories on the anterior surface of the medulla oblongata. They are composed of projection fibre bundles which originate in the precentral gyrus of the cerebrum and the majority of fibres decussate (cross over to the contralateral side).

Defer, deferent[ial]. The vas deferens carries seminal fluid from the testis.

Originally, the letter symbolised the triangular opening into a tent! The delta of a river usually has this Δ shape as, not surprisingly, do the muscle and ligament.

Dentine, dentist, dentition, denture. The dens is the odontoid (tooth-shaped) process. Although attached to the axis, it actually represents the body of the atlas.

Part of the hippocampal complex.

Anatomical Names	Latin/Greek or Other Origins	Examples
Dermis, dermal	**Derma**: [Gr] *skin, pelt, leather*	Dermis
Dermatome	**Derma + tomos**: [Gr] *slice, cut, a part cut out*	Dermatome
Diaphragm, diaphragmatic	**Dia-**: [Gr] *across*; **phragma**: [Gr] *fence*	Diaphragm Costodiaphragmatic *recess*
Digiti, digitorum, digitation	**Digitus**: [L] *finger, toe*	Flexor digiti minimi m
		Flexor digitorum longus m
Distal	**Distare**: [L] *to be distant, apart, different*	Distal
Diverticulum	**Diverticulum**: [L] *by-road, diversion, digression*	Diverticulum ilei
Dorsum, dorsal, dorsi	**Dorsum**: [L] *back*	Dorsum
		Latissimus dorsi m
		Dorsal root
Duodenum, duodenal	**Duodeni**: [L] *numbered or divided in units of 12*	Duodenum

Notes, Links and Non-Anatomical Usages

Dermatology, dermatitis, pachyderms (a group of mammals with thick skin, including elephants, rhinos and...politicians?). Dermis is now just part of the skin, the other part being the epidermis (on the dermis). By the way, did you know that skin is the largest organ of the body?

Dermatome (a strip of skin cut out to be supplied by nerves from a particular spinal level), myotome (a mass of skeletal muscle supplied by a particular spinal level), microtome (an instrument for cutting small slices).

The diaphragm separates the thoracic and abdominal cavities. An area of pleural cavity between costal and diaphragmatic pleurae into which the lung expands during inspiration.

Digital, digitigrade (toe-walker, a group of animals which, like horses, walk on their toes), prestidigitation (sleight of hand with nimble fingers!), inter-digitating (interlocking like the fingers of 2 hands). The flexor digiti minimi m (flexor of the little finger) is an intrinsic muscle of the hand supplied by the deep branch of the ulnar n. What is the name of the eminence under which this and other little finger mm lie?

The long flexor of the 4 lateral toes. It runs from the tibia distal to the soleal line and runs to the distal phalanx of a toe. It also helps to plantar flex at the ankle joint. Nerve supply?

Distance, distant. The distal end of a limb is the part furthest from the limb root.

Diversion, diverticulitis. The diverticulum ilei (or Meckel's diverticulum) is an embryological remnant which may contain ectopic gastric tissue.

Dorsiflexion. Dorsal and posterior are used interchangeably.

The very broad muscle of the back is innervated by the thoracodorsal n and is a medial rotator, extensor and adductor of the arm at the shoulder joint. Where does it insert on the humerus?

Contains afferent nerve fibres passing information to the spinal cord. It bears a swelling, the dorsal root ganglion, which contains unipolar neurons with bifurcating dendro-axonal processes.

Duodenum (this is traditionally 12 finger-widths long), duodecimal.

Anatomical Names	Latin/Greek or Other Origins	Examples
Dura, dural	**Durus**: [L] *hard, stiff, lasting*	Dura mater
		Dural reflections
		Epidural

E.

Anatomical Names	Latin/Greek or Other Origins	Examples
Efferent	**Efferens**: [L] *carrying away*	Efferent nerve Efferent lymphatic
Epididymis	**Epi-**: [Gr] *near, upon*; **didymos**: [Gr] *twin, testicle*	Epididymis
Epiglottis, epiglottic	**Epi-**: [Gr] *near, upon*; **glossa/glotta**: [Gr] *tongue*	Epiglottis Aryepiglottic folds
Epiploic	**Epiploon**: [Gr] *bowels, membrane*	Epiploic foramen
Ethmoid, ethmoidal	**Ethmos**: [Gr] *sieve*; **eidos**: [Gr] *shape, form*	Ethmoid bone Sphenoethmoidal recess
Eversion, evertors	**E[x]-**: [L] *out*; **vertere**: [L] *to turn*	Eversion Evertor mm

Durable (hard-wearing, lasting), endurance (ability to last), duration (the period over which something endures), Durex (tradename for a presumably hard-wearing condom), obdurate (refusing to change an opinion or action, hard-hearted). The dura mater is the tough, outermost layer of the 3 meninges covering brain and spinal cord.

A term used to describe the arrangement of the dura mater within the cranial cavity.

Literally, on or around the dura mater. Such an injection is made into the space surrounding the dura mater, usually of the spinal cord.

Efferent – carrying away from (e.g. the CNS, an organ or a lymph node).

Epididymis (near the testicle) – a firm mass of coiled tubes about 6 metres long lying posterior to the testis. It has a head (caput), body (corpus) and tail (cauda). If there's anyone reading this by the name of Thomas, your name comes from an Aramaic word-root for twin. And that's not a load of ….!

It is near the tongue.

Run from arytenoid to epiglottic cartilages.

Epiploon is equivalent to omentum [L]. The epiploic foramen is the communication between the lesser and greater peritoneal sacs. Its anterior wall is the free edge of the lesser omentum which contains 3 important vessels: bile duct on the right, hepatic a on the left and portal v behind and between.

So… the cribriform plate of the ethmoid bone is the sieve-like plate of the sieve bone!

A small region of the nasal cavity above the superior concha and into which opens the sphenoidal and, maybe, posterior ethmoidal air sinuses.

Eversion of the foot involves turning the sole of the foot outwards (laterally). At what joints does this occur?

The set of muscles which produce eversion of the foot, i.e. peroneus longus m and …?

Anatomical Names	Latin/Greek or Other Origins	Examples
Extension, extensor	**Extendere**: [L] *extend, straighten, stretch out*	Extension Extensor muscles
Externus	**Externus**: [L] *external, outward, foreign, strange*	Obliquus externus m

F.

Anatomical Names	Latin/Greek or Other Origins	Examples
Falx, falciform	**Falx**: [L] *sickle, scythe*	Falx cerebri
		Falciform ligament
Fascia, fasciae, fascial	**Fascia**: [L] *band, bandage*	Superficial/deep fascia
Fascicle, fasciculus, fasciculi, fascicular	**Fasciculus**: [L] *little bundle*	Fasciculus
Fauces	**Fauces**: [L] *throat, jaws, pass, straits, isthmus*	Fauces
Femur, femoral, femoris	**Femur**: [L] *thigh*	Femur
		Femoral artery
		Biceps femoris m

Notes, Links and Non-Anatomical Usages

Extend, extent, extensive, extenuate. Extension usually involves straightening out the joint and is brought about by the action of extensor mm.

The external oblique mm of the abdomen have fibres running in the same direction as the fingers when the hands are in trouser pockets, i.e. downwards and medially. Its aponeurosis helps to form which important ligament running between the anterior superior iliac spine and the pubic tubercle?

Plasmodium falciparum (the infectious agent of the most severe form of malaria is sickle-bearing), falcon (because the beak is sickle-shaped?). The falx cerebri is the sickle-shape fold of dura mater which contains the sagittal dural venous sinuses and helps limit side-to-side and antero-posterior movement of the brain within the cranial cavity.

The sickle-shaped ligament is a peritoneal fold running from the umbilicus up to the portal area of the liver. In its free border is the ligamentum teres, the remains of the umbilical v which delivered oxygenated blood to the fetus in utero.

Fascia or facia. Superficial fascia is synonymous with the histological term, hypodermis. In the abdominal wall, it is divisible into a superficial fatty layer and a deep membranous layer. The latter forms the superficial layer of the superficial perineal pouch.

The gracile and cuneate fasciculi are ascending tracts of nerve fibres in the posterior part of the medulla oblongata.

Fauces (area between oral cavity and pharynx). The fauces are bounded on each side by mucosal ridges, the palatoglossal folds. Between these and the more posterior palatopharyngeal folds, the palatine tonsils normally lie.

Femur (bone of thigh), femoral (relating to the femur or thigh).

The femoral a enters the thigh behind the inguinal lig at a point midway between the anterior superior iliac spine and the pubic symphysis. The pulse of the artery can be palpated at this site by pressing gently backwards against pectineus m and the superior pubic ramus.

'The two-headed thigh muscle'. So-called to distinguish it from biceps brachii m.

Anatomical Names	Latin/Greek or Other Origins	Examples
Fenestra, fenestrae	**Fenestra**: [L] *window, wall opening*	Fenestra cochleae
		Fenestra vestibuli
Fibula, fibular	**Fibula**: [L] *clasp, buckle, brooch, pin*	Fibula
		Fibular
Filum, fila	**Filum**: [L] *thread, string, fibre*	Filum terminale
Fimbria, fimbriae	**Fimbria**: [L] *fringe, border*	Fimbria of the uterine tube
Flexion, flexor	**Flexio**: [L] *bending*	Flexion
		Flexor muscles
Flocculus, floccular	**Floccus**: [L] *flock, lock of unspun wool*	Flocculonodular lobe
Folium, folia, foliate	**Folium**: [L] *leaf*	Folia of the cerebellum
		Foliate papillae

Notes, Links and Non-Anatomical Usages

Fenestrated (such capillaries have openings in their endothelium), defenestration (to throw someone out of a window!). The fenestrae cochleae and vestibuli are two windows in the medial wall of the tympanic cavity. The former is closed by a membrane and looks on the scala tympani of the cochlea. The fenestra vestibuli leads into the vestibule of the inner ear and the base of the stapes fits snugly into it so that vibrations of the stapes may be transmitted to the inner ear.

Fibula (a pin – if you look at the tibia and fibula together, especially in a small mammal such as a rabbit, they look like a clasp with the tibia being the catch and the fibula the pin).

Fibular is sometimes used to mean on the lateral side (of the leg or ankle). The peroneal mm are sometimes called the fibular mm.

Filament (thin wire thread in a light-bulb), fillet (a thin boneless strip of meat), filaria (a group of parasitic nematodes also known as the thread-worms!). In adults, the spinal cord ends at L1-L2 vertebral level. From this point, a prolongation of the pia mater, the filum terminale (the terminal thread), descends to attach to the coccyx.

Fimbriated (fringed). The fimbriae of the uterine tube arise from the infundibulum. One fimbria, the ovarian fimbria, is longer than the others and is applied to the tubal pole of the ovary.

Flex, flexible. Flexion usually involves bending at a joint. It is effected by flexor mm. In the case of the ankle, there is plantar flexion and dorsiflexion. Plantar flexion is assisted by long toe flexors but dorsiflexion is assisted by toe extensors.

Flocculent (aggregated in woolly, cloudlike masses), a flock mattress is stuffed with wool waste or torn-up cloth, flock wallpaper bears powdered wool or cloth. The flocculonodular node of the cerebellum is on its inferior aspect and is composed of 2 lateral tufted outgrowths, the flocculi, and a single midline nodule. Together they are concerned with maintaining balance (equilibration).

Foliage, folic acid (found in green leaves), portfolio (a case for carrying important papers). The cerebellar surface is divided into folds (folia; singular folium) and grooves (fissures) which are the counterparts of cerebral gyri and sulci respectively.

The mucosa of the superior surface of the tongue bears taste, touch and pressure receptors. Foliate papillae are reddish, leaf-like and tend to lie at the sides at the junction of its oral and pharyngeal parts. They contain taste buds.

Anatomical Names	Latin/Greek or Other Origins	Examples
Follicle, follicular	**Folliculus**: [L] *little bag*	Lymphoid follicle
		Hair follicle
Foramen, foramina	**Foramen**: [L] *hole, opening, aperture*	Foramen magnum
		Foramen lacerum
		Foramen ovale
		Foramen rotundum
		Foramen spinosum
Fornix, fornices	**Fornix**: [L] *arch, vault, brothel situated therein*	Fornix
Fossa, fossae	**Fossa**: [L] *ditch, trench, recess*	Fossa ovalis
		Cranial fossae
Fovea	**Fovea**: [L] *pit, snare*	Fovea centralis
		Pterygoid fovea
Frenulum	**Frenum**: [L] *bridle, bit, band*	Frenulum (of tongue, lips, prepuce, clitoris)
Frontal, frontalis	**Frons**: [L] *front, forehead*	Frontal bone

Lymph node cortex contains dense aggregates of lymphocytes (lymphoid follicles). Follicles may be primary or secondary and the lymphocytes are mainly B with some helper T cells.

The epidermal pit through which the hair shaft grows to reach the surface of the skin.

Foraminifera (protozoa with shells having numerous openings in them). The foramen magnum is just that – a big hole.

The mangled or torn hole, transmitting what?

The oval hole, transmitting what?

The rounded hole, transmitting what?

The spine-related hole because of its nearness to the spine of the sphenoid bone.

Fornication (Roman prostitutes entertained clients under the arches of the Colosseum and other buildings!). The fornices of the vagina encircle the vaginal cervix and provide important sites via which surrounding pelvic structures may be palpated.

Fossil (often dug up), fossorial (having a digging habit, like a mole). The fossa ovalis is a depression in the inferior part of the interatrial septum of the heart. It is the remnant of the foramen ovale which shunted blood away from the pulmonary circulation in the fetal heart.

There are anterior, middle and posterior cranial fossae. Which brain regions are found in each?

On the posterior of the retina is an oval macula lutea (yellow spot) which is the area of greatest visual acuity. It has a central depression, the fovea centralis (central pit).

A triangular depression on the anterior of the neck of the mandible into which the lateral pterygoid m is inserted. What are the origins of this muscle?

In all cases, the frenulum forms a fold which checks the range of movement of the structure to which it attaches.

Front, frontispiece. A frontal plane passes vertically like a coronal plane (see above). The frontal bone is the bone of the forehead. With which other skull bones does it articulate?

Anatomical Names	Latin/Greek or Other Origins	Examples
		Occipitofrontalis m
Fundus	**Fundus**: [L] *foundation, bottom*	Fundus (of bladder, stomach, uterus)
G.		
Ganglion, ganglionic	**Ganglion**: [Gr] *tumour, swelling*	Dorsal root ganglion
		Ganglion impar
		Pre- or post-ganglionic
Gastric, gastro-	**Gastrikos**: [Gr] *related to the stomach*	Gastric vv
		Epigastric region
		Gastrocnemius m
		Digastricus m
Gemellus, gemelli	**Gemellus**: [L] *little twin;* **geminus**: [L] *twin*	Gemelli mm
Genicular, geniculate	**Geniculatus**: [L] *jointed, having knots;* **geniculum**: [L] *little knee*	Genicular branches of the obturator n
		Geniculate ganglion of facial n
Genioid, genio-	**Geneion**: [Gr] *chin*	Genioid tubercles

Notes, Links and Non-Anatomical Usages

A muscle of facial expression with occipital and frontal bellies joined by a tough aponeurosis of the scalp (the epicranial aponeurosis). Contraction of the frontal bellies on both sides raises the eyebrows.

Profound (deep), the fundus is the base of an organ when viewed from the traditional surgical approach. Foundation, fund, fundament (also a humorous term for the buttocks or bottom!).

Ganglion – a swelling caused by a collection of neurons. The dorsal root ganglion is a sensory ganglion associated with the dorsal root.

Impar: [L]: different, unequal. The ganglion impar is formed anterior to the coccyx by the meeting of the 2 sympathetic trunks. It is single and unpaired and, therefore, different from other ganglia.

Terms used to distinguish fibres running to a ganglion or from a ganglion.

Gastrointestinal, gastronomic, gastrula. Left and right gastric vv drain the stomach and lesser omentum and empty into the portal v. Where do the short gastric vv drain and empty?

The epigastric region or epigastrium (near the stomach) is the upper middle region of the anterior abdominal wall. The lower middle region is the hypogastrium (below the stomach).

Gastrocnemius m (belly-leg, i.e. calf muscle). What are its attachments?

Has 2 bellies!

The gemelli twins are the superior and inferior gemellus mm. These very small muscles are accessory lateral rotators of the hip joint. The constellation Gemini contains the heavenly twins, Castor and Pollux.

Genicular branches of the obturator n pass to the knee joint (together with other branches from which named nerves?).

This ganglion is found on the site (called the geniculum) where the facial n alters its course. The ganglion is sensory and is associated with which special sense?

Genial (related to the chin). The genioid tubercles lie on the posterior aspect of the mental area of the mandible and are sometimes called the mental (mentum: [L] chin) spines or tubercles. They are attachment sites for important muscles. Here's one now!

Glossary 2   **57**

Anatomical Names	Latin/Greek or Other Origins	Examples
		Genioglossus m
Genu	**Genu**: [L] *knee*	Genu of corpus callosum
Gland, glans	**Glans**: [L] *acorn, nut, bullet;* **glandula**: [L] a term for *swollen glands in the neck*	Glans penis
		Salivary glands
Glenoid, glenoidal, gleno-	**Glene**: [Gr] *socket;* **eidos**: [Gr] *shape, form*	Glenoid fossa/cavity
		Glenoidal labrum
		Glenohumeral lig
Glossal, glosso-, -glossus, glottis, glottidis	**Glossa** or **glotta**: [Gr] *tongue*	Hypoglossal n (cranial XII)
		Glossopharyngeal n (cranial IX)
		Hyoglossus m
		Epiglottis
		Rima glottidis
Gluteus, gluteal	**Gloutos**: [Gr] *buttock, rump*	Gluteus maximus m
		Gluteal lines
Gracilis	**Gracilis**: [L] *slender, lean*	Gracilis m
Gubernaculum	**Gubernaculum**: [L] *helm, rudder, tiller;* **gubernator**: [L] *governor*	Gubernaculum testis

Notes, Links and Non-Anatomical Usages

Pulls the tongue forwards and out of the mouth.

Genuflect (to pray or go down on bended knee), genuine (when a Roman child was born, it was the practice for the father to claim it as his own by putting it on his knee!). The genu of the corpus callosum is at its anterior pole where, on a sagittal section, it looks as though the white matter bends. The posterior pole of the corpus callosum is called what?

The glans penis is the swelling at the distal end of the penis. Its skin is removed during circumcision ("The unkindest cut of all?").

The paired parotid, submandibular and sublingual salivary glands.

The glenoid fossa is an articular socket for the humeral head.

The labrum is the fibrocartilaginous rim of the glenoid fossa.

These are weak ligaments reinforcing the joint capsule anteriorly.

Glossary, glottal. The hypoglossal n supplies all intrinsic and most extrinsic mm of the tongue. What are the exceptions?

Leaves the cranial cavity through which foramen? It supplies taste to the posterior 2/3 of the tongue and contributes to the pharyngeal plexus. It innervates only one skeletal muscle. Which one?

Runs from hyoid bone to tongue and depresses the latter.

Lies near the tongue (but see rima glottidis below).

The rima glottidis is the gap between the vocal cords.

Gluteus maximus is the largest of 3 gluteal mm. The others are?

Again, there are 3 and they are associated with the origins of gluteal mm. Can you recall them?

Gracile (= slender). Homo gracilis was of slender build. The gracilis m is a long, slender muscle which is part of the adductor group of the thigh. So what is its innervation?

The gubernaculum testis 'steers' the testis in its descent from the posterior abdominal wall, via the inguinal canal, and into the scrotum. In the USA, gubernatorial elections decide who the state governors will be.

Anatomical Names	Latin/Greek or Other Origins	Examples
Gyrus, gyri	**Gyrus**: [L] *circle, coil, ring*	Precentral gyrus

H.

Hamate	**Hamus**: [L] *hook*	Hamate bone
Hamulus	**Hamulus**: [L] *little hook*	Pterygoid hamulus
Hiatus	**Hiatus**: [L] *gap, opening*	Adductor hiatus
		Hiatus semilunaris
Hilum, hilus, hilar	**Hilum**: [L] *the scar on a seed where it joins its stalk*	Hilum (of liver, lung, spleen, etc)
Hippocampus, hippocampal	**Hippos**: [Gr] *horse*; **kampos**: [Gr] *sea creature*	Hippocampus
Hymen	**Hymen**: [Gr, L] *God of Marriage*, [Gr] *membrane*	Hymen
Hyoid, hyo-	**Hyo-**: [Gr] *related to U, the letter upsilon*; **eidos**: [Gr] *shape, form*	Hyoid bone
		Hyoglossus m
Hypophysis, hypophyseal	**Hypo-**: [Gr] *below, down*; **physis**: [Gr] *growth*	Hypophysis
Hypothenar	See Thenar below	

I.

Ileum, ileal, ilei, ileo-	**Ile**: [L] *gut*; **ilia**: [L] *entrails, loins*	Ileum

Notes, Links and Non-Anatomical Usages

Gyrate (spin round), gyroscope. The precentral gyrus of the cerebrum is the motor area and lies anterior to the central sulcus. What gyrus lies immediately behind the sulcus?

The hamate bone is a carpal bone with a hook to which the flexor retinaculum attaches.

Hamulus – used to describe hook-like appendages. The pterygoid hamulus is a small hook-shaped piece of bone hanging from the inferior of the medial pterygoid plate. You should be able to palpate this at the posterolateral angle of your own hard palate!

Hiatus hernia is herniation through an anatomical gap. The adductor hiatus is a gap in the adductor magnus tendon at which the femoral a becomes the popliteal a. Does anything else pass through this hiatus?

A groove on the medial wall of the nasal cavity.

The hilum (or hilus) of an organ is the site at which its vessels (mainly blood vessels) enter and leave, so you should be able to appreciate the analogy.

The hippocampus of the forebrain was named because of its resemblance, in a coronal section, to a seahorse (generic name Hippocampus).

Hymeneal (relating to marriage), hymenoptera (insects, e.g. bees and wasps, with 2 pairs of membranous wings).

The hyoid bone is U-shaped with the body and 2 lesser horns anteriorly and 2 greater horns posteriorly.

The hyoglossus m runs from the hyoid bone to the tongue. It is an extrinsic muscle of the tongue which depresses it (nerve supply?).

Diaphysis, epiphysis, metaphysis. The hypophysis cerebri (to give its full name) is a downgrowth or offshoot of the cerebrum commonly known as the pituitary gland.

Ileostomy, ileitis. Here, ileum refers to entrails (bowels, guts).

Anatomical Names	Latin/Greek or Other Origins	Examples
		Ileal aa
		Ileocolic aa
		Diverticulum ilei
Iliac, ilium, ilio-	**Ilia**: [L] *entrails, loins*	Ilium (iliac bone)
		Iliolumbar lig
Ima	**Ima**: supposedly from [L]: *lowest*	Thyroidea ima a
Incus	**Incus**: [L] *anvil*	Incus
Index, indicis	**Index**: [L] *fore-finger, informer, witness, spy*	Index finger
		Extensor indicis m
		Radialis indicis a
Infundibulum, infundibular	**Infundibulum**: [L] *funnel, funnel-shaped passage*	Infundibulum (of uterine tube, hypothalamus)
Inguinal, inguinalis	**Inguen**: [L] *groin*	Inguinal region
		Inguinal lig
		Falx inguinalis
Internus	**Internus**: [L] *internal, civil, domestic*	Obliquus internus m

Branches of the superior mesenteric a.

Branches of the superior mesenteric a.

Meckel's diverticulum: in 2% of subjects, 2 feet from the ileocolic junction and about 2 inches long! It may contain ectopic acid-secreting tissue and mimic symptoms of appendicitis.

Here, the term ilium refers to the loins. The ilium is at the inferior end of the anatomical loins (running from twelfth rib to iliac crest) but superolateral to the poetic loins (the private parts).

The iliolumbar lig runs from the transverse process of the L5 vertebra to the iliac crest. It is the inferior attachment of the quadratus lumborum m.

The lowest (and smallest and least constant) of the arteries supplying the thyroid gland. It may arise from the right common carotid, subclavian or internal thoracic aa or from the aorta. What are the more important sources of arterial supply to the thyroid gland?

Incuse (the design stamped on a coin). The incus is one of the 3 auditory ossicles, malleus (hammer), incus (anvil) and stapes (stirrup). All easily identifiable by their shapes!

Indicate (to point with the index finger!), indicative.

An extensor of the index finger. Supplied by the radial n.

The artery on the lateral (radial) side of the index finger. It arises from the radial a in the palm as it passes through the first dorsal interosseous m.

Infundibular. Whether part of the uterine tube or hypothalamus, it is still funnel-shaped.

The region where the thigh joins the abdomen.

The inrolled inferior margin of the aponeurosis of the external oblique m which helps define the inguinal canal.

Another name for the sickle-shaped conjoint tendon of the fused fibres of internal oblique m and transversus abdominis m which runs to the pubic tubercle, crest and pecten.

Internal. Obliquus internus (internal oblique) mm of the abdomen have fibres running at right angles to those of external oblique mm.

Anatomical Names	Latin/Greek or Other Origins	Examples
Intimi, intima	**Intimus**: [L] *innermost, deepest*	Intercostales intimi mm
		Tunica intima
Inversion, invertors	**In-**: [L] *in, inwards*; **vertere**: [L] *to turn*	Inversion
		Invertor mm
Ipsilateral	**Ipse**: [L] *self, same*; **latus**: [L] *side*	Ipsilateral
Ischium, ischial, ischio-	See Sciatic below	

J.

Jejunum, jejunal	**Jejunus**: [L] *empty, hungry*	Jejunum
		Jejunal vv
Jugular	**Jugulum**: [L] *neck, throat, collar;* **jugum**: [L] *yoke*	Jugular notch

L.

Labium, labia, labial	**Labium**: [L] *lip*	Labium major
Labyrinth, labyrinthine	**Labyrinthos**: [Gr] *maze, labyrinth*	Labyrinth
		Labyrinthine aa

Notes, Links and Non-Anatomical Usages

Intimacy, intimate. The intercostales intimi mm are sometimes called the innermost intercostal mm. Like external and internal intercostal mm, those of a given intercostal space are supplied by the corresponding intercostal n but between which pair of muscles does the nerve run?

The innermost layer of a blood vessel wall composed of squamous endothelial cells. What are the middle and outer layers called and what are their principal tissue types?

Inversion of the foot is when the sole turns inwards.

The invertors of the foot include tibialis anterior m (nerve supply?) and … ?

Ipsilateral (on the same side) is in contrast to contralateral. Two Latin expressions still in use: ipse dixit (he himself said it – refers to an unproven or dogmatic assertion); ipso facto (by that very fact).

Jejune (naïve, insipid, dull). Jejunum is actually an abbreviation of intestinum jejunum (empty intestine) derived from the observation that often, after death, the jejunum is empty.

Drain into the superior mesenteric vv and then into which vein?

Jugulate (to slit the throat!), subjugate (put under the yoke). Yoke itself comes from the word-root jugum. A yoke is a wooden frame attached to the neck of oxen or worn on a person's shoulders to carry things. The jugular notch is an alternative name for the suprasternal notch. Just above it, the two anterior jugular vv are connected to each other by a vein called the jugular arch.

Labials (sounds produced by using the lips). The major labia are the larger of the 2 sets of lips associated with the female external genitalia.

The labyrinth of the ear has bony and membranous parts and is a complex subserving hearing and balance.

The artery supplies the inner ear and is usually a branch of the basilar a or the anterior inferior cerebellar a and it accompanies which cranial nn into the internal acoustic (auditory) meatus?

Anatomical Names	Latin/Greek or Other Origins	Examples
Labrum	**Labrum**: [L] *lip, edge, rim*	Glenoidal labrum
Lacrimal	**Lacrima[e]**: [L] *tear[s]*	Lacrimal gland
Lacuna, lacunae, lacunar	**Lacuna**: [L] *pit, hole, chasm;* **lacus**: [L] *lake, pond*	Osteocyte lacuna(e) Lacunar ligament
Lambda, lambdoid	**Lambda**: [Gr] *Greek letter* λ; **eidos**: [Gr] *shape*	Lambda Lambdoid suture
Lamina, laminae, laminar	**Lamina**: [L] *plate, leaf, blade, thin piece of metal*	Cricoid lamina Thyroid lamina
Lateral, lateralis	**Latus**: [L] *side, flank*	Lateral head of triceps m Vastus lateralis m
Latissimus	**Latus**: [L] *broad, extensive, wide, copious;* **latissimus**: [L] *very broad, wide*	Latissimus dorsi m

Labret (any body-piercing ornament attached to a lip). The glenoidal labrum is the rim of the glenoid fossa of the scapula.

Lacrimation (tear flow, i.e. weeping), lacrimatory (something which causes lacrimation, e.g. a freshly-sliced onion, a good joke or a kick in the ...!). The gland is situated in the superolateral part of the orbit but lacrimal fluid drains from a duct found at the medial angle of the eye. So tears run across the eye downwards and medially.

Lagoon (laguna: [It,Sp]) is from this word-root as is the word lake. Each osteocyte (bone cell) dwells in a small cavity called a lacuna but the cells remain multiply interconnected by cell processes.

The lacunar lig is at the medial end of the inguinal lig and may be so-called because of the space between the inguinal lig and the pelvic bone or because its free edge is the medial margin of the femoral ring which leads into the femoral canal.

The area of the skull where the sagittal and lambdoid sutures meet (so, corresponds to the apex of the letter λ). In the neonate, the parietal and occipital bones are partially unfused and the posterior fontanelle is found at this site.

The lambdoid suture between the occipital and parietal bones is lambda-shaped.

Laminated (laminated wood is made of several layers bonded together), laminin (a protein of the basal lamina). The cricoid lamina is the flat posterior plate of cartilage. The thyroid laminae on both sides meet anteriorly at an angle which is sharper in males than in females. And that's why the "Adam's apple" is more prominent in males!

The lateral head of the triceps m arises from the upper and lateral half of the posterior humeral shaft above the radial (or spiral) groove. A common tendon for all 3 heads of triceps inserts on the olecranon process of the ulna.

This muscle arises from the intertrochanteric line, base of the greater trochanter and linea aspera of the femur. It inserts into the tendon of quadriceps femoris m and, hence, into the patella. What is its nerve supply?

Defining position on the Earth requires angles of latitude and longitude. The latissimus dorsi m is the very broad muscle of the back. It has an origin from the dense thoracolumbar fascia and inserts on the humerus at the intertubercular groove. What are its actions and nerve supply?

Anatomical Names	Latin/Greek or Other Origins	Examples
Lentiform	**Lens**: [L] *lentil*; **forma**: [L] *shape*	Lentiform nucleus
Levator	**Elevare**: [L] *to lift, raise*	Levator scapulae m
Lieno-	**Lien**: [L] *spleen*	Lienorenal lig
Ligament, ligamentum	**Ligamen**: [L] *band, tie*	Ligamentum nuchae
Limbus, limbic	**Limbus**: [L] *border, fringe, hem, stripe, band*	Limbic lobe
		Limbic system
Lingual	**Lingua**: [L] *tongue, language*	Lingual n
Lingula, lingulae	**Lingula**: [L] *little tongue*	Lingula
Lumbar, lumborum, lumbo-	**Lumbus**: [L] *loin*	Lumbar plexus
		Quadratus lumborum m

Notes, Links and Non-Anatomical Usages

Lens (named because of its shape resemblance to a lentil), lenticular or lentoid (biconvex, like a lentil). The lentiform nucleus is part of the corpus striatum and comprises a medial and pale globus pallidus (pale globe) and a darker lateral putamen (meaning shell or husk).

Elevate, elevator (a lift), levitation. Levator mm generally raise (e.g. levator scapulae raises the scapula) or support (levator ani supports pelvic viscera).

The lienorenal lig is a peritoneal reflection from the left kidney to the spleen. The splenic a runs within its layers.

Ligament (ties bones together), ligand, ligature. The ligamentum nuchae (ligament of the nape of the neck) runs from the occiput down to the spine of C7 vertebra. It binds cervical spinous processes together and acts as an attachment site for cervical musculature.

Limbo (the borders of Hell!). The limbic lobe is a collective term often used to describe the cingulate gyrus + parahippocampal gyrus + uncus. These cerebral structures border the corpus callosum and third ventricle.

The limbic system is a complex which includes the limbic lobe and medial parts of the frontal lobe interconnected with the hypothalamus, thalamus, basal ganglia and other deep nuclei. It is involved in emotional expression and experience.

Linguistics, language (via langue: [Fr] tongue). Ironically, the phrase lingua franca (French tongue – referring to a common language used by people with different Mother tongues) is Italian and not French! The lingual n (a branch of which cranial n?) supplies taste to the anterior 2/3rds of the tongue.

The lingula of the mandible is a tongue-like bony projection which lies next to the mandibular foramen and to which attaches the sphenomandibular lig. The lingulae of the lung and cerebellum are also tongue-like.

Lumbar puncture, lumbago (low back pain). Anatomically, the loins extend from the false ribs to the iliac crest. A loin chop includes the psoas major m (psoa: [Gr] loin muscle) and part of the adjacent lumbar vertebra. The lumbar plexus is associated with ventral primary rami of spinal nn L1-L4 supplemented by a branch of T12. What named nerves arise from this plexus?

A quadrate muscle attaching to the twelfth rib, iliolumbar lig and iliac crest.

Anatomical Names	Latin/Greek or Other Origins	Examples
		Lumbosacral trunk
Lumbrical	**Lumbricus**: [L] *worm*	Lumbrical mm
Lunate, lunar, lunaris	**Luna**: [L] *moon*	Lunate bone
		Semilunar valves
		Hiatus semilunaris

M.

Anatomical Names	Latin/Greek or Other Origins	Examples
Macula	**Macula**: [L] *spot, blemish*	Macula lutea
Malleolus, malleolar	**Malleolus**: [L] *small hammer*	Medial malleolus
Malleus	**Malleus**: [L] *hammer, mallet*	Malleus
Mammary	**Mamma**: [L] *breast, teat, mother*	Mammary gland
Mam[m]illary	**Mammilla**: [L] *breast, teat*	Ma[m]illary bodies

Branches of the 4th and 5th lumbar spinal nn of the lumbar plexus which descend on the pelvic sacrum to join the sacral plexus.

Lumbricus terrestris is the common earthworm. The lumbrical mm of each hand (4 in number) are worm-like muscles. They originate on tendons of flexor digitorum profundus mm and insert on lateral sides of metacarpophalangeal joints of digits 2-5 (so what are their actions?). Their innervations mirror the nerve supplies of flexor digitorum profundus m: the medial 2 lumbricals are supplied by the ulnar n and the lateral 2 by the median n.

Lunar, lunate, lunatic (whose sanity was believed to be affected by the lunar cycle!). The lunate bone is crescent-shaped so the term doesn't refer just to the full moon.

Here, it's a half moon shape that is being referred to.

A curved groove on the medial wall of the nasal cavity created, in part, by the bulge of the ethmoidal bulla.

Immaculate (literally, spotless). The macula lutea (yellow spot) of the retina is a yellowish spot with a depression at its centre (the fovea centralis) which is the region of greatest visual acuity.

The medial malleolus (a tibial prominence) is slightly superior to the lateral (a fibular prominence). Both malleoli resemble little hammer-heads. Behind the medial malleolus are several important structures which can be remembered as Tom, Dick and Harry moving posteriorly (Tom is tibialis posterior tendon, Dick is flexor digitorum longus tendon and Harry is flexor hallucis longus tendon. Where do the posterior tibial a and tibial n lie with respect to these tendons?).

Mallet, malleable (literally, hammerable). The malleus is one of the auditory ossicles in the tympanic cavity. It is caused to vibrate by movements of the tympanic membrane. What muscle damps down movements of the malleus and what is its innervation?

Ma, mam, mam[m]a, mammary, mammal. All derive from this basic wordroot and the child's first sounds "ma-ma".

The mammillary bodies are 2 small, breast-like protruberances on the brain base at the upper border of the pons. In front of them is the pituitary stalk or infundibulum.

Anatomical Names	Latin/Greek or Other Origins	Examples
Mandible, mandibular	**Mandere**: [L] *to chew*	Mandible
		Submandibular gland
Manubrium	**Manubrium**: [L] *hilt, handle;* **manus**: [L] *hand*	Manubrium
Masseter, masseteric	**Masein**: [Gr] *to chew*	Masseter m
		Masseteric n
Mastication	**Masticare**: [L] *to chew*	Muscles of mastication
Mastoid	**Mastos**: [Gr] *breast;* **eidos**: [Gr] *shape*	Mastoid process
Mater, matrix	**Mater**: [L] *mother* (hence *protector* connotation); **matrix**: [L] *a female kept for breeding* (hence, *womb*)	Dura, arachnoid, pia mater
Maxilla, maxillae, maxillary	**Maxilla**: [L] *jawbone, jaw*	Maxilla
		Maxillary n
Meatus, meati	**Meatus**: [L] way, channel	External auditory meatus
		Nasal meati

Notes, Links and Non-Anatomical Usages

The mandible is the bone of the lower jaw – the jaw free to move during chewing! What muscles are required for this action?

A salivary gland situated below the mandible. What is its secretomotor innervation?

Short for manubrium sterni (the handle of the sternum). Manual, manicure, manifesto, manufacture (handmade), manuscript (handwritten).

The masseter is a muscle of mastication (chewing).

Supplies the muscle and arises from which division of cranial V?

Masticatory. Mastic is an aromatic gum from the mastic tree and is used to flavour chewing gum!

Mastitis, mastectomy, mastodon (breast-like tooth – an extinct elephant-like animal with nipple-like tubercles on the crowns of its molar teeth). The mastoid process is part of the temporal bone and, after about the first postnatal year, is a breast-like projection lying posterior to the internal acoustic meatus. Why is it poorly developed in neonates?

Mater (Victorian term for mother; the 3 meninges help to protect the brain and spinal cord), maternal, matron, matriculate, matrimony. A matrix may also be supportive or nutritive (like the womb), e.g. extracellular matrix.

The upper jawbone. The bone is less dense than that of the mandible making it easier for dentists to anaesthetise the teeth and gums simultaneously. In the mandible, teeth and gums must be anaesthetised by separate injections.

This nerve is a branch of cranial V. It is exclusively sensory. What is its area of supply?

The external auditory (or acoustic) meatus is the channel running from the auricle to the tympanic membrane. It slopes downwards anteromedially and contains ceruminous glands secreting wax. How might this wax (or other irritation of the mucosa) trigger a cough reflex?

The superior, middle and inferior meati are the channels running anteroposteriorly between the nasal conchae and floor of the nasal cavity. What structures open into each meatus?

Anatomical Names	Latin/Greek or Other Origins	Examples
Medial, median	**Medius**: [L] *middle, in the middle, middling*	Medial
		Median n
Mediastinum	**Mediastinum**: [L] *a menial (slave), his/her quarters*	Mediastinum
Medulla, medullary	**Medulla**: [L] *marrow, pith, inmost part* (related to medius and can imply *'in the midline'*)	Adrenal medulla Medulla oblongata
Meninx, meninges, meningeal	**Meninx**: [Gr] *membrane*	The meninges
		Middle meningeal a
Mentum, mental	**Mentum**: [L] *chin*	Mental n
Mesentery, mesenteric	**Mesos**: [Gr] *middle*; **enteron**: [Gr] *gut, intestine*	The mesentery
		Superior mesenteric a
Molar	**Molarius**: [L] *concerned with milling or grinding*; **molaris**: [L] *related to a mill-stone*	Molar teeth
Mucosa, mucosae, mucosal, mucous	**Mucosus**: [L] *slimy, mucous*	Mucosa
Muscle, muscular[is]	**Musculus**: [L] *little mouse, muscle*	Muscle
		Muscularis mucosae

Notes, Links and Non-Anatomical Usages

Medium, medieval, mediocre (literally, half way up the mountain, but meaning of moderate quality!). Medial structures lie closer to the body's midline. A median structure lies in the midline.

The median n of the upper limb arises from the lateral cord of the brachial plexus and runs roughly down the middle of the anterior compartments of the upper limb. It supplies muscles in the anterior compartments of the forearm and hand. What is its sensory innervation?

The mediastinum is a set of regions into which the thoracic cavity can be divided. What are the different regions called?

The adrenal medulla is the inmost part; the medulla oblongata is in the midline.

The meninges are a set of 3 membranes surrounding the brain and spinal cord (dura, arachnoid and pia mater).

The largest of the meningeal aa. It enters the cranial cavity through which foramen?

Not to be confused with mental from mens: [L] mind. The mental foramen of the mandible transmits which nerve? Of what nerve is it a terminal branch?

The mesentery slings the abdominal foregut to the posterior abdominal wall and is found in the middle of the intestinal mass.

The arterial supply of the midgut.

Molar (a tooth for grinding food).

Mucus, mucin, mucopolysaccharide.

Muscular. Muscle was named by analogy to the jerky, darting movements of a mouse.

The smooth muscle layer associated with a mucosa (e.g. of the small intestine).

Anatomical Names	Latin/Greek or Other Origins	Examples
N.		
Navicular	**Navicula**: [L] *little boat*	Navicular bone
Nephron, nephric	**Nephros**: [Gr] *kidney*	Nephron
		Mesonephric duct
Node, nodular	**Nodus**: [L] *knot, tie, swelling*	Lymph node
		Flocculonodular lobe
Nucleus	**Nucleus**: [L] *kernel, nut, inside*	Nucleus pulposus
O.		
Obturator	**Obturare**: [L] *to close, stop up, block off, obstruct*	Obturator foramen
Occiput, occipital	**Occiput**: [L] *back of head*	Occiput
		Occipital condyle
Ocular, oculi, oculo-	**Oculus**: [L] *eye*	Extraocular mm
		Orbicularis oculi m
		Oculomotor n (cranial III)

Navy, naval, navigation. The disarticulated bone can be seen to resemble a little boat.

Nephric (meaning the same as renal), nephrology, nephritis, nephropathy. The nephron is the main functional unit of the kidney, comprising the renal corpuscle and its associated uriniferous tubule.

During embryological development 3 kidney systems develop sequentially, the middle of which is the mesonephros (middle kidney). The excretory tubules first appear in the mesonephros. At one end, they form the renal corpuscle and, at the other, they enter the collecting (mesonephric or Wolffian) duct.

Nodule, nodose.

Phylogenetically, an ancient part of the cerebellum. See Flocculus above.

Nuclear, nucleated, nucleolus, nucleic acid, nuclease, etc. The nucleus pulposus is the elastic, central part of an intervertebral disc. Inordinate pressure may cause this to be squeezed through the outer annulus fibrosus to produce a ruptured or herniated disc. This may impinge on the spinal cord causing pain, numbness or loss of muscle function.

To obturate (to obstruct). The obturator foramen, in life, is partially closed by the obturator membrane through which passes the obturator n.

The occipital bone articulates with the atlas and has some important openings: the foramen magnum and anterior condylar (or hypoglossal) canal.

The occipital condyles articulate with superior facets on the atlas and these atlanto-occipital joints allow what movements?

Ocular (also used to describe the eyepiece of a microscope), oculist. The extraocular (outside the eye) mm are the extrinsic muscles which move the eye within the orbit. What are their names, actions and innervations?

The orbicularis oculi m (encircling muscle of the eye) is a muscle of facial expression allowing you to close the eyelids and 'screw up' your eyes. As you know, it is supplied by the facial (cranial VII) n.

The oculomotor (eye-moving) m supplies which extraocular mm?

Anatomical Names	Latin/Greek or Other Origins	Examples
Odontoid, -odontal	**Odon**: [Gr] *tooth*; **eidos**: [Gr] *shape*	Odontoid process
		Periodontal lig
Olecranon	**Olene**: [Gr] *elbow*; **kranion**: [Gr] *head*	Olecranon
Olfaction, olfactory	**Olfactus**: [L] *odour, sense of smell*	Olfaction
		Olfactory n (cranial I)
Omentum, omental	**Omentum**: [L] *bowels, fat, membrane, caul*	Greater omentum
		Omental bursa
Omohyoid	**Omos**: [Gr] *humerus, shoulder* (see Hyoid above)	Omohyoid m
Ophthalmic	**Ophthalmos**: [Gr] *eye*	Ophthalmic a
Optic	**Optikos**: [Gr] *related to sight*	Optic n
Oral, oris, oro-	**Oralis**: [L] *of the mouth*	Oral cavity
		Orbicularis oris m
		Oropharynx
Otic, oto-	**Otikos**: [Gr] *related to the ear*	Otic ganglion
		Otocyst

Notes, Links and Non-Anatomical Usages

Odontology, orthodontist (makes sure you have 'straight teeth'). The odontoid process is shaped like a tooth and its alternative name (dens: [L] tooth) proves it!

The periodontal ligament, or periodontal membrane, 'surrounds the tooth'. It is a dense fibrous connective tissue supporting the tooth in its socket and lying between the alveolar bone and the dental cement.

The head of the elbow – actually the bony prominence at the proximal end of the ulna.

Olfaction is the special sense of smell.

Helps to connect the olfactory mucosa of the upper nasal cavity to the olfactory cortex ('smell brain').

The greater omentum is suspended from the greater curvature of the stomach and is supplied by which arteries?

This lesser peritoneal sac lies posterior to the lesser omentum and communicates with the greater sac via the epiploic foramen.

The omohyoid m (nerve supply?) joins the shoulder (actually the scapular notch on the superior scapular border) to the hyoid bone. Like the digastricus m, it has 2 bellies. Recall that the acr[o]-omion (acromion) forms the tip of the shoulder.

Ophthalmology. The ophthalmic a arises from the internal carotid a in the middle cranial fossa and enters the orbit via which opening?

Optical, optician. The optic n is cranial n II.

Oration (what comes out of the mouth!).

A muscle of facial expression which compresses the lips.

The mouth part of the pharynx, as distinct from the nose (nasopharynx) and larynx (laryngopharynx) parts.

Otorhinolaryngology (ear, nose and throat), parotid (near the ear), otitis media (inflammation of the middle ear).

The inner ear rudiment.

Anatomical Names	Latin/Greek or Other Origins	Examples
P.		
Palatine, palati[ni], palato-	**Palatum**: [L] *palate*	Palate
		Palatine nn
		Levator veli palati[ni] m
		Palatopharyngeus m
Palpation	**Palpare**: [L] *to touch gently*	Palpation
Pampiniform	**Pampinus**: [L] *tendril, vine-shoot*	Pampiniform venous plexus
Papilla, papillae, papillary	**Papilla**: [L] *nipple, teat, breast*	Greater duodenal papilla
		Papillary mm
Parietal	**Paries**: [L] *wall*	Parietal (bones, peritoneum, pleura, etc)
Parotid	**Para**: [Gr] *near*, **otos**: [Gr] *ear*	Parotid gland
Patella, patellar	**Patella**: [L] *small dish, plate, pan*	Patella
		Infrapatellar bursa

The palate comes hard or soft, like a boiled egg.

Greater and lesser palatine nn and nasopalatine nn supply the hard and soft palate. From which cranial openings do they emerge?

Raises the soft palate during swallowing.

A vertical pharyngeal muscle which also assists swallowing. How?

Palpate (to inspect anatomically by gentle touch), palpable (able to be felt or touched).

The pampiniform plexus associated with the testicular blood supply is a complex network of veins which are tributaries of the testicular v and closely associated with the testicular a (like tendrils around the stem of a vine). There is countercurrent heat exchange between artery and venous plexus which helps maintain a lower testicular temperature.

Papilloma (a wart-like growth). However, the colloquial term pap (nipple, teat, breast) is ON in origin and is probably imitative of the lip-smacking sounds at suckling. The greater duodenal papilla is where the bile and main pancreatic ducts converge to enter the 2nd part of the duodenum on its posteromedial wall.

Extensions of myocardium into the ventricular cavities which help close the atrioventricular valves.

Parietal literally means related to the walls and all anatomical structures with this name are exactly that.

Parotid (situated near the external ear). The gland lies anterior to the mastoid process, external ear and sternocleidomastoid m and passes superficial and deep to the ramus of the mandible. These, and other, salivary glands swell in mumps patients. Swelling of the parotid gland is particularly painful because its fibrous capsule is especially strong superficially.

Hence, Spanish 'paella' which is cooked in a large shallow pan. The patella (bone of the knee-cap) resembles an inverted dish or small bowl.

Subcutaneous and deep infrapatellar bursae are associated with the knee joint (patella and patellar lig). They may become enlarged after prolonged kneeling. Do they communicate with the knee joint cavity?

Anatomical Names	Latin/Greek or Other Origins	Examples
Pecten, pectineal, pectinati	**Pecten**: [L] *comb, rake*	Pecten pubis, pecten ani
		Pectineus m
		Musculi pectinati
Pectoral[is], pectoris	**Pectus**: [L] *breast (= chest)*	Pectoralis major m
		Clavipectoral fascia
Peduncle, peduncular	**Pedunculus**: [L] *small foot, stalk*	Cerebral peduncles
		Interpeduncular fossa
Pelvis, pelvic	**Pelvis**: [L] *basin*	Pelvis
		Pelvic diaphragm
Peritoneum, peritoneal	**Peri**: [Gr] *around*; **tonos**: [Gr] *stretched*	Peritoneum
Peroneus, peroneal	**Perone**: [Gr] *fibula, pin*	Peroneus longus m

Notes, Links and Non-Anatomical Usages

The symbol for the Shell Oil Company is a pectinate mollusc! Areas with this name usually have some comb-like appearance or relationship.

A muscle of the thigh helping to form the floor of the femoral triangle. It arises from the pecten pubis of the superior pubic ramus and inserts just below the lesser trochanter of the femur. It is usually supplied by the femoral n but may also be supplied by which other nerve?

These muscles are found in the wall of the right atrium of the heart. The back of the comb is the crista terminalis and the teeth of the comb are the musculi pectinati.

Angina pectoris (chest pain). The pectoralis major m has 2 heads: clavicular and sternocostal. These fibres collectively insert where?

Deep fascia investing the pectoral minor and subclavius mm and attaching to the axillary fascia and clavicle. The part between the upper border of pectoralis minor m and the clavicle is sometimes called the costocoracoid membrane and is pierced by the cephalic v, thoracoacromial a and lateral pectoral n.

The pedunculate oak is the common or English oak. It produces stalked acorns. The cerebral peduncles join the cerebrum to the midbrain. Each has a ventral crus cerebri and dorsal tegmentum separated by substantia nigra.

An area associated with the optic chiasma, tuber cinereum and pituitary stalk, mammillary bodies and posterior perforated substance. The crura cerebri of the cerebral peduncles form the caudolateral boundaries of this fossa.

Pelvimetry (obstetrical measurement of pelvic dimensions). The pelvic region is made of the pelvic and sacral bones and is divided into an upper or false pelvis (false because this basin has no anterior wall) and a lower or true pelvis.

The muscular sling for pelvic viscera comprising the levator ani and coccygeus mm.

Peritoneum stretches around the abdominal cavity and viscera. Peritonitis (inflammation of peritoneum).

Peroneal means the same as fibular. This muscle is an evertor of the foot and supplied by the superficial branch of the common peroneal n.

Anatomical Names	Latin/Greek or Other Origins	Examples
		Common peroneal n
Pes, pedis	**Pes**: [L] *foot*	Pes planus
		Dorsalis pedis a
Petrous, petrosal	**Petra**: [L] rock, stone	Petrous part of temporal bone
		Petrosal sinuses
Phalanx, phalanges, phalangeal	**Phalanx**: [Gr] *bone of finger or toe*	Proximal phalanx The phalanges
		Metacarpo-phalangeal joint
Phrenic	**Phrenikos**: [Gr] *related to the diaphragm*	Phrenic n
		Musculophrenic a
Pia, pial	**Pia**: [L] *tender, delicate*	Pia mater
Pisiform	**Pisum**: [L] *pea*; **forma**: [L] *shape*	Pisiform bone
Placenta	**Plakoeis**: [Gr] *flat cake*; **placenta**: [L] *pancake*	Placenta

Notes, Links and Non-Anatomical Usages

The nerve passes into, and divides on, the lateral (fibular) side of the leg into deep and superficial branches.

Pedal, pedestrian, pedicure, pedicel. Pes planus is flat foot.

A lower limb pulse site on the dorsum of the foot. Situated where precisely?

Petrify (turn to stone), Peter the Rock (the most steadfast of the disciples of Jesus. Actually, the name Peter means 'the rock' anyway!). The petrous part of the temporal bone is its densest and helps to protect delicate internal structures like the inner ear.

Dural venous sinuses which help drain the cavernous sinus.

Phalangeal. In ancient Macedonia, Alexander the Great inherited from his father, Philip, an invincible fighting unit, a line of infantry in close ranks, called a phalanx. The thumb and big toe have 2 phalanges (proximal, distal) but all other fingers and toes have an additional intermediate or middle phalanx.

These joints are articulations between metacarpal and proximal phalangeal bones.

Phrenic (in Greek, also relates to the mind, hence phrenology. This is because they thought that the mind resided in the diaphragm. No, I can't see the logic either!).

The internal thoracic a in the sixth intercostal space divides into 2 branches. The musculophrenic a is one and it supplies the periphery of the diaphragm and the adjacent thoracic wall. What is the other branch and what does it supply?

The innermost and most delicate of the meninges. It is the layer which accompanies the small blood vessels as they enter the substance of the brain.

A pea-shaped carpal bone. The proper name for the garden pea is Pisum sativum (satisfying pea). The old word for pea, pease (as in the nursery rhyme "Pease pudding hot, pease pudding cold...etc"), is from the same word-root.

Aptly named if you have seen one just delivered!

Anatomical Names	Latin/Greek or Other Origins	Examples
Plantar, plantaris	**Planta**: [L] *sole of the foot*	Long plantar lig
		Plantaris m
Platysma	**Platys**: [Gr] *flat, wide, broad, ample*	Platysma m
Pleura, pleurae, pleural	**Pleura**: [Gr] *side or rib*	Parietal pleura
		Pleural cavity
Plexus	**Plexus**: [L] *plaited, interwoven, braided*	Sacral plexus
Pollex, pollicis	**Pollex**: [L] *thumb*	Pollex
		Flexor pollicis longus m
Pons, pontine	**Pons**: [L] *bridge, drawbridge*	Pons
		Pontine cistern
Popliteus, popliteal	**Poples**: [L] *knee*	Popliteal fossa
		Popliteus m
Porta, portal, porto-	**Porta**: [L] *door, entrance, outlet*	Porta hepatis

Plantigrade (walking on the sole of the foot, like humans). The long plantar lig strengthens the calcaneocuboid joint inferiorly.

A vestigial muscle not always present. It is associated with the lateral head of gastrocnemius m and inserts on the medial side of the posterior calcaneum. What do you think would be its motor nerve supply?

Plato (was broad-shouldered), platyhelminths (flatworms), platypus (broad of foot). The platysma m is subcutaneous and a muscle of facial expression used when grimacing. Nerve supply?

Parietal pleura lines the ribcage, pleurisy (inflammation of pleura).

The potential space between parietal and visceral pleurae.

Complex, perplex. Plexuses are formed from nerves or veins. The sacral plexus of nerves is formed by the lumbosacral trunk (L4, L5) and ventral rami of S1-S4. What are its branches? A sacral venous plexus joins lateral sacral vv (tributaries of the internal iliac vv) which accompany the lateral sacral aa.

Pollex, in Latin, also meant big toe which is now called the hallux.

The long flexor of the thumb is supplied by which nerve?

The pons bridges the brain hemispheres. Pontoon bridge! Pontefract (broken bridge) in Yorkshire is the traditional site of UK manufacture of liquorice sweets. Pont l'Evêque (bishop's bridge) in Normandy is the site of manufacture of a favourite cheese of mine.

Contains cerebrospinal fluid and lies anterior to the pons. The basilar a runs through the cistern in the midline.

The popliteal fossa lies behind the knee joint. What are its boundaries?

The muscle forms part of the floor of the popliteal fossa. It arises from the lateral femoral condyle and the arcuate popliteal lig and inserts on the tibia above the soleal line. It unlocks the knee prior to flexion. What movement does unlocking involve?

Airport, portal (door in poetry), portcullis (sliding door), portico. The porta hepatis (portal area of the liver) is the hilum where vessels enter (hepatic a, portal v) and leave (bile duct).

Anatomical Names	Latin/Greek or Other Origins	Examples
		Portosystemic anastomosis
Profunda, profundus	**Profundus**: [L] *deep, profound*	Profunda femoris a
		Flexor digitorum profundus m
Pronation, pronator	**Pronus**: [L] *bent, inclined towards, bowing*	Pronation
		Pronator teres m
Protraction, protractor	**Pro-**: [L] *forwards*; **trahere**: [L] *to draw, pull*	Protraction
Protrusion, protrusor	**Pro-**: [L] *forwards*; **trudere**: [L] *to thrust*	Protrusion
Proximal	**Proxime**: [L] *nearest, next, very close to*	Proximal
Pterion	**Pteron**: [Gr] *wing, anything wing-like*	Pterion
Pterygoid	**Pteron**: [Gr] *wing, anything wing-like*	Lateral pterygoid plate

Notes, Links and Non-Anatomical Usages

Occurs between portal and systemic venous circulations. In portal hypertension, where are the commonest sites of venous distension for diagnostic purposes?

Profound (spatially or intellectually deep). Remember that deep in Anatomy always means further away from the skin surface. The profunda femoris a is a deep muscular branch of the femoral a. Its own branches contribute to which important anastomoses?

The deep flexor of the fingers. At what joints does this muscle produce flexion?

Prone (meaning lying face down or inclined to), pronate. Pronation in the forearm involves rotation of the radius and its movement relative to the ulna so that the palm of the hand faces posteriorly. The radius turns anteromedially to lie obliquely across the ulna. Which movement is stronger, pronation or supination?

One of the 2 main pronators of the forearm, the other being pronator quadratus m. Both are supplied by the median n. What other forearm muscle may assist in pronation/supination?

Protracted, extract, tractor. In protraction of the upper limb (as when extending the reach), the scapula is pulled anteriorly. By what muscles?

Protrude. Protrusion of the mandible is brought about by the pterygoid mm, particularly the lateral pterygoid mm. These are supplied by the mandibular division of cranial n V.

Approximate (close to), proximity. In a limb, proximal structures are closer to the root of the limb. Proxima Centauri is the closest star to our solar system.

Pterodactyl (a reptile with wings supported by an elongated digit), pterygotes (the winged insects). The pterion is on the lateral aspect of the skull and represents the smallest circle which contains the suture at which the frontal, parietal, sphenoid and squamous temporal bones meet. The name may derive from the fact that the sphenoid component is from the greater wing of the sphenoid. The bone at this site is liable to fracture because it is naturally thin and, in addition, eroded internally by which artery?

The pterygoid plates are wing-like postero-inferior extensions of the sphenoid bone which, itself, has lesser and greater wings! The lateral plate provides origins for both the lateral and medial pterygoid mm.

Anatomical Names	Latin/Greek or Other Origins	Examples
Ptosis	**Ptosis**: [Gr] *drooping, falling*	Ptosis
Pudenda, pudendal	**Pudendus**: [L] *shameful, disgraceful*	Pudenda
		Pudendal n
Pulmonary	**Pulmo**: [L] *lung*	Pulmonary a
Pulvinar	**Pulvinar**: [L] *sofa, bed, couch (all cushioned)*	Pulvinar
Putamen	**Putamen**: [L] *shell (of fruit), husk, peelings, clippings, waste*	Putamen
Pylorus, pyloric	**Pyloros**: [Gr] *gatekeeper*	Pylorus Pyloric sphincter

Q.

Quadrate, quadratus	**Quadratus**: [L] *square, quadrangular*	Quadrate tubercle Quadratus femoris m
Quadriceps	**Quadriceps**: [L] *four-headed*	Quadriceps femoris m

R.

Radius, radial[is]	**Radius**: [L] *stick, rod, poke, weaver's shuttle*	Radius

Notes, Links and Non-Anatomical Usages

Ptosis of the upper eyelid is a diagnostic sign of what? (Name the muscles and nerves.) Apoptosis (falling away) is loss of cells by programmed cell death.

Pudenda (the external genitalia – short for pudenda membra meaning, literally, the parts to be ashamed of! We still speak of them as the "naughty bits"). An impudent person originally was one who had no shame or displayed his/her genitals in public – a streaker?

One of the main terminal branches of the sacral plexus (S2-S4). It runs between the piriformis and coccygeus mm to enter the greater sciatic foramen. It then passes behind the sacrospinous lig and into the lesser sciatic foramen, thereby bypassing the pelvic diaphragm. It enters the pudendal canal, a fascial sheath on the lateral wall of the ischiorectal fossa. What does the nerve supply?

Pulmonates (molluscs, including slugs and snails, in which the mantle cavity is modified to act as a lung). Remember that not all arteries convey oxygenated blood. The pulmonary aa convey deoxygenated blood from the right ventricle to the lungs.

The pulvinar is so-called because this part of the thalamus projects like a cushion or knob.

Part of the lentiform nucleus. Maybe named because, in a frontal slice, the whole lentiform nucleus looks like odd scraps?

The pyloric sphincter guards the pylorus (gate between stomach and duodenum).

Quadrat. The quadrate tubercle of the intertrochanteric crest of the femur provides attachment for the quadratus femoris m. What are the actions of this muscle? Also, the liver has a quadrate lobe.

Of course, you know that the 4 heads are rectus femoris, vastus lateralis, medius and intermedius mm.

Radius (rod or stick is not a bad description of the bone), radial. The bone is on the lateral side of the forearm and moves with respect to the ulna during pronation and supination.

Anatomical Names	Latin/Greek or Other Origins	Examples
		Radial a
		Flexor carpi radialis m
Ramus, rami	**Ramus**: [L] *branch, twig*	Ramus of the mandible
		Rami communicantes
Raphe	**Raphe**: [Gr] *stitching, seam*	Raphe of the pharynx
Rectum, rectus, recto-	**Rectus**: [L] *straight, regular*	Rectum
		Rectus abdominis m
		Rectouterine pouch
Renal	**Renes**: [L] *kidneys*	Renal vv
		Adrenal (suprarenal) gland

Notes, Links and Non-Anatomical Usages

Arises from the brachial a in the cubital fossa. Its pulse may be palpated where?

The flexor of the wrist on the radial (= lateral) side. It arises from the common flexor origin on the medial epicondyle of the humerus and inserts on the palmar aspect of metacarpal bases 2 and 3. It is supplied by the median n. What are its antagonists and synergists in movements at the wrist?

Ramify (to form branches), ramification. The ramus of the mandible extends from the angle and runs upwards to branch into the condylar and coronoid processes.

Ventral rami of spinal nn T12-L2 have branches called white rami communicantes which pass to ganglia on the sympathetic trunk. Axons from ganglion cells pass from the trunk and rejoin the spinal nn as grey rami communicantes. Fibres in white rami are myelinated and preganglionic. Those in grey rami are non-myelinated and postganglionic. To what structures are the postganglionic sympathetic fibres in the spinal nn distributed?

A raphe tends to be a midline seam where sheets of tissue (usually muscle) meet. That of the pharynx provides attachment for the constrictor mm.

Rectum (hopefully, you stay regular!), rectal, rectangular (right-angled), rectify (to put straight), rectilinear (in a straight line), rectitude.

The 'straight muscle of the abdomen'. The strap-like muscles on either side run down the anterior abdominal wall from lower thoracic cage to pubis and are separated by the linea alba. They are supplied by ventral rami of T7-T12 spinal nn and enclosed in the rectus sheath. What are the actions of the muscle and the contributors to the anterior and posterior parts of the rectus sheath?

The rectouterine pouch (of Douglas) is a peritoneal reflection from the posterior of the uterus on to the rectum.

Adrenal, adrenaline, suprarenal, renin. The renal vv drain into the IVC but are of unequal length. On which side is the renal v shorter?

Adrenal means 'near the kidney' and, interestingly, American English borrowed the Greek for this (epinephron) in order to derive epinephrine which is the American equivalent of adrenaline.

Anatomical Names	Latin/Greek or Other Origins	Examples
Rete	**Rete**: [L] *net, fishing-net*	Rete testis
Reticulum, reticular	**Reticulum**: [L] *little net*	Endoplasmic reticulum
		Reticular formation
Retinaculum	**Retinaculum**: [L] *stay, tie*	Flexor retinaculum
Retraction, retractor	**Retro-**: [L] *backwards*; **trahere**: [L] *to draw, pull*	Retraction
Rhomboid	**Rhomboid**: [Gr] *rhombus-like in shape*	Rhomboid major m
Rima	**Rima**: [L] *crack, chink, fissure*	Rima glottidis
Rostrum, rostral	**Rostrum**: [L] *bill, beak, snout, anything projecting*	Rostrum of the corpus callosum
Rotation, rotator	**Rotare**: [L] *to turn (in a circle)*	Rotation (medial, lateral)

Notes, Links and Non-Anatomical Usages

Rete (used to describe complexes of small vessels), retiarius (a type of Roman gladiator who fought with a net and trident), retina. The rete testis is a network of anastomosing tubes lying between the seminiferous tubules of the testis and the efferent tubules of the caput epididymis.

Reticle, reticule (once a woman's bag or purse), reticulocyte (immature red cell with vestiges of protein synthetic machinery stainable with basic dyes and appearing as a reticulum). Endoplasmic reticulum is a subcellular organelle of interconnected tubules and cisternae involved in protein synthesis and export.

A complex network of nerve fibres and grey matter scattered throughout the medulla oblongata, pons and midbrain. Sometimes called the reticular activating system, it is concerned with stimulating the cerebral cortex into a state of arousal or wakefulness. Decreased activity results in sleep. I hope your reticular formation is currently active!

A retinaculum retains tendons, or other structures, in place. The flexor retinaculum of the wrist constrains flexor tendons and stops them bowstringing during wrist flexion. What other structures pass superior and deep to this retinaculum?

Retract (to withdraw). Latissimus dorsi m is a powerful retractor of the humerus. What muscles retract the scapula?

A rhombus is a four-sided, oblique-angled parallelogram with equal sides. In a rhomboid, adjacent sides are of unequal length. The rhomboid major mm are rhomboidal muscles which help brace the shoulders by retracting the scapulae. They are supplied by the dorsal scapular nn but what are their attachments?

The rima glottidis is the gap between the vocal cords. The glottidis element refers to the tongue but, anatomically, strictly to the area of the vocal cords. Rima [L] is not to be confused with rima: [OE] rim, border, edge.

Rostrum, rostra (a platform for a speaker, conductor – in Roman times, the public platform was decorated with the ramming beaks from defeated enemy ships!). The rostrum of the corpus callosum projects anteriorly to the genu and downwards to the lamina terminalis (anterior wall of third ventricle). Rostral (like cephalic) is also used to indicate nearer to the head, as opposed to the tail (caudal), end of the body.

Rotate, rotary, rotor, rotifer (a multicellular invertebrate with a ciliated wheel-like organ used for feeding and locomotion). Recall that the axis of rotation of a long bone does not always correspond to the long axis of the bone.

Anatomical Names	Latin/Greek or Other Origins	Examples
		Rotator cuff mm
S.		
Saccule, sacculus	**Sacculus**: [L] *little sac*	Saccule or sacculus
Sacrum, sacral, sacro-	**Sacrum**: [L] *sacred thing, solemn site, sacrifice*	Sacrum
		Sacral promontory
		Sacroiliac joint
Sagittal	**Sagitta**: [L] *arrow*	Sagittal suture
Salpinx, salpingo-	**Salpinx**: [Gr] *tube, trumpet*	Salpinx
		Mesosalpinx
		Salpingo-pharyngeus m
Saphenous	Origin obscure: probably **saphena**: [ML] *vein*, or **saphene**: [Gr] *clear, obvious, plain*, but possibly **safin**: [Arab] *hidden, silent, secret*!	Great saphenous v
Sartorius	**Sartor**: [L] *tailor*	Sartorius m

Muscles (subscapularis, supraspinatus, infraspinatus, teres major) whose tendons help stabilise the shoulder joint.

The term sacculus is used to describe various anatomical sac-like spaces in the internal ear, larynx and elsewhere.

Short for os sacrum (holy bone, because the Greeks and Romans thought that it housed the soul!), sacred, sacrifice.

The sacral promontory is the anterior projecting rim of the upper surface of the first sacral vertebra. In the anatomical position, the centre of gravity of the body lies just below this promontory.

A synovial joint between the sacral and iliac articular surfaces. In infants, the joint is plane but, in adults, movement is restricted by interlocking ridges and valleys. The range of movement increases in pregnant females.

Sagittarius (the Archer constellation). A sagittal plane runs vertically through the body in the midline and in an anteroposterior direction. Hence the name sagittal suture.

Salpiglossis (a plant with trumpet-like flowers), The term salpinx may refer to the uterine tube which, when blocked, requires surgical intervention, salpingostomy.

The mesosalpinx is the mesentery of the uterine tube.

Here, salpinx refers to the auditory tube. The muscle is supplied by the pharyngeal plexus but what are its attachments and actions?

So, possibly, the great venous vein or obvious vein (when it is varicose?) or hidden vein (because it lies medially and, normally, is not varicose?).

Sartorial (related to a tailor or to tailoring). Traditionally, a tailor sits on a floor or bench with legs akimbo, i.e. with lower limbs flexed at hip and knee, and thigh abducted and laterally rotated. All actions of the sartorius m!

Anatomical Names	Latin/Greek or Other Origins	Examples
Scala	**Scala**: [L] *ladder, staircase, spiral*	Scala tympani, media, vestibuli
Scaphoid	**Scaphoid**: [Gr] *keel-shaped*	Scaphoid fossa, bone
Sciatic, ischium, ischial, ischio-	**Ischion**: [Gr] *hip*	Sciatic n
		Greater sciatic foramen
		Ischial tuberosity
		Ischiocavernosus m
Sella	**Sella**: [L] *saddle*	Sella turcica
Septum, septa, septal, septo-	**Septum**: [L] *fence, enclosure*	Nasal septum Septal cartilages
		Septomarginal trabecula
Serratus	**Serratus**: [L] *like the teeth of a saw*	Serratus anterior m
Sesamoid	**Sesamon**: [Gr] *sesame, sesame seed*	Sesamoid bones

Notes, Links and Non-Anatomical Usages

Scalable (able to be climbed, like a ladder or staircase), scalariform cells (water-conveying plant cells with thickened, ladder-like walls), scale (a measuring scale or ruler is analogous to a ladder). The scala tympani (lower), media (middle) and vestibuli (upper) are spaces within the spiral cochlea of the inner ear.

At the base of the medial pterygoid plate is a hollow just like the keel of a boat! The carpal bone also has boaty features.

Sciatica (pain associated with the nerve). The sciatic n is a major terminal branch of the sacral plexus. What is the link between this nerve and foot-drop?

Lies above the level of the ischial spine and sacrospinous lig. What structures pass through it?

The ischial tuberosity is a roughened area of bone on the ischium which provides attachment for several muscles. Which ones?

This is one of them, a perineal muscle of the superficial perineal pouch which runs from the ischial tuberosity to the crus penis (male) or crus clitoridis (female). It helps compress the crus and so maintain erection of the penis or clitoris. The muscle is supplied by which branch of the pudendal n?

The 'turkish saddle' (on account of its shape) or hypophyseal fossa (because it contains the hypophysis or pituitary gland) is a depression in the sphenoid bone lying above the sphenoidal air sinus.

Septal cartilages and bone help to make the nasal septum which separates the 2 nasal cavities.

A band of muscular and conducting tissue running across the right ventricle from the interventricular septum to the base of the anterior papillary m.

Serratus anterior inserts on ribs 2-9 and interdigitates with attachments of external oblique m. The interdigitations look serrated, like the teeth of a saw!

Sesamoid bones are 'seeded' and grow within tendons (e.g. the pisiform bone in flexor carpi ulnaris tendon and the patella in quadriceps femoris tendon).

Anatomical Names	Latin/Greek or Other Origins	Examples
Sigmoid, sigmoidal	**Sigmoid**: [Gr] *S-shaped* (the equivalent letter S is called sigma in Greek)	Sigmoid sinus, colon
Sinus, sinu-	**Sinus**: [L] *hollow, cavity*	Oblique sinus
		Paranasal air sinuses
		Sinuatrial node
Skull	**Skalle**: [ON] *skull*; **skål**: [ON] *drinking bowl*	Skull
Soleus, soleal	**Solea**: [L] *sole of the foot*	Soleus m
		Soleal line
Somatic	**Soma**: [Gr] *the body*	Somatic
Sphenoid, sphenoidal, spheno-	**Sphen**: [Gr] *wedge*; **eidos**: [Gr] *shape, form*	Sphenoid bone
		Sphenoidal air sinus
		Sphenomandibular lig
Spinal	**Spina**: [L] *thorn, spine, prickle, backbone*	Spinal cord (medulla)

Notes, Links and Non-Anatomical Usages

Sigma, sigmoidal. All sigmoidal structures display an S-shape or a sinuous course. A sigmoidoscope is used to view internally the sigmoid colon.

Sinusitis, sinusoid (sinus-like). The oblique sinus of the heart is a J-shaped space behind the left atrium created by pericardial reflections. The limb of the J contains the IVC and right pulmonary vv whilst the foot contains the left pulmonary vv.

A set of cavities within skull bones lined by respiratory mucosa and communicating with the nasal cavities. What are their names and sites of drainage into the nasal cavity?

The pacemaker of the heart initiates the cardiac cycle and sets the basic frequency. Its cells are situated in the wall of the right atrium near the SVC opening and adjacent crista terminalis.

When Norsemen drink, they say "skål" which means "cheers". It may be that the drinking bowl was made originally from a skullcap of some animal. Is it just chance that people who drink to excess are described as being 'out of their skulls'?

Soleus m is a calf muscle which runs down towards the sole of the foot (actually inserting on the calcaneum) and produces plantar flexion at the ankle.

A line of attachment of the soleus m to the superior part of the posterior aspect of the tibia.

Somatotype (classification of body type by physique or build). In Anatomy, somatic is used in 2 main senses: to contrast with visceral (related to organs) or with germinal (related to germ cells). For example, cranial nn contain 4 main types of nerve fibre: somatic afferent, visceral afferent, somatic efferent and visceral efferent.

The bone is a complicated structure resembling 2 pairs of wings. It sits wedged into the skull by surrounding bones.

Opens and drains where?

A rather vestigial structure extending between which particular bits of the sphenoid bone and mandible?

Spine. The spinal cord does not extend the whole length of the vertebral column. In adults, it terminates at what level?

Anatomical Names	Latin/Greek or Other Origins	Examples
Spinosum	**Spinosus**: [L] *thorny, prickly, spiny*	Foramen spinosum
Splanchnic	**Splanchna**: [Gr] *the entrails, innards*	Splanchnic nn
Stapes, stapedius	**Stapes**: [L] *stirrup*	Stapes Stapedius m
Stellate	**Stella**: [L] *star*	Stellate ganglion
Stria, striae, striate[d], striatum	**Stria**: [L] *groove, stripe*	Olfactory stria Striate cortex Striated muscle Corpus striatum
Stroma, stromal	**Stroma**: [Gr] *couch, bed, mattress, layer*	Stroma
Styloid, stylo-	**Stylos**: [Gr] *column*	Styloid process Styloglossus m Stylomastoid foramen

Notes, Links and Non-Anatomical Usages

Spinose (= spiny). The foramen spinosum is just anteromedial to the spine of the sphenoid bone. What artery does it transmit?

Splanchnic sometimes means the same as visceral but refers to the organs in the abdomen rather than in general. There are sympathetic splanchnic nn (associated with thoracic spinal levels T5-T12) and parasympathetic splanchnic nn (sacral levels S2-S4). What viscera do they innervate?

Stapes (the ear ossicle is a perfect little stirrup!), stapedial.

The stapedius m damps down excessive movements of the stapedius caused by loud sounds. If this muscle, or its nerve supply, are affected then acoustic disturbances may follow. Damage to which cranial n may result in hyperacusia?

Stellar, constellation (all stars together – just like Oscars night!). The stellate ganglion is near the neck of the first rib and is formed by the fusion of the inferior cervical and first thoracic ganglia of the sympathetic trunk.

Lateral and medial olfactory striae arise from each olfactory tract just in front of the anterior perforated substance of the brain and optic chiasma.

A frontal section through the junction of the calcarine and parieto-occipital sulci of the occipital cortex reveals a stripe of white matter embedded in the grey matter. The stripe reflects the organisation of the visual cortex and this area is called the striate cortex.

So-called because the striped appearance (due to the regular organisation of actin and myosin filaments) is particularly noticeable histologically in this type of muscle.

Grey matter extends in strips between putamen and caudate nucleus and appears striated in a frontal slice.

The term stroma is often used to refer to the connective tissue component of an organ or part thereof.

The styloid process is shaped like a little column.

The muscle attaches to the styloid process and is the smallest and shortest of 3 muscles which do so. What are their nerve supplies?

A small foramen between the styloid and mastoid processes of the temporal bone. Part of the facial n leaves this foramen and radiates to supply the various muscles of facial expression.

Anatomical Names	Latin/Greek or Other Origins	Examples
Sulcus, sulci	**Sulcus**: [L] *furrow, rut, little ditch, groove*	Cingulate sulcus
		Sulcus terminalis (tongue and right atrium)
Superficial[is]	**Superficies**: [L] *surface*; **superficialis**: [L] *related to the surface*	Flexor digitorum superficialis m
Supination, supinator	**Supinus**: [L] *lying on the back*	Supination
		Supinator m
Sural	**Sura**: [L] *calf of the leg*	Sural n
Symphysis	**Syn**: [Gr] *together;* **physis**: [Gr] *growth*	Pubic symphysis
Synergist, synergism	**Syn**: [Gr] *together,* **ergon**: [Gr] *work*	Synergistic muscle

T.

Anatomical Names	Latin/Greek or Other Origins	Examples
Taenia, taeniae	**Taenia**: [L] *band, ribbon, narrow strip*	Taenia[e] coli
Talus, talar, tali, talo-	**Talus**: [L] *ankle*	Talus
		Tibiotalar lig
		Sustentaculum tali

Sulcate (grooved). The cingulate sulcus partially girdles the corpus callosum on the medial surface of the cerebrum.

Both grooves act as boundaries. In the tongue, it is between the embryologically distinct anterior and posterior parts; in the atrium, it is between different embryological parts of the right atrium.

Remember that, in Anatomy, superficial always signifies closer to the skin surface. A superficial person is "only skin deep"…or less! Flexor digitorum superficialis m is a superficial finger flexor. It is supplied by the median n. Does it flex anything else apart from the finger joints?

Supine, supinate. In supination, the forearm bones lie roughly parallel to each other.

One of the supinators of the forearm. It is supplied by the radial n and acts best when the elbow is extended. What acts best as a supinator in flexion at the elbow?

The sural n (spinal levels L5-S2) arises from the tibial division of the sciatic n but is joined by a communicating branch of the common peroneal n. What is its distribution?

When the 2 pubic bones meet and fuse together, they make the pubic symphysis. Symphyseal or symphysial.

Synergy, synergistic, energy (that which does work). Synergistic muscles act together to produce a given movement.

Taeniasis (tapeworm infestation), taeniafuge (a drug for getting rid of tapeworms). Taeniae coli are 3 thin strips of smooth muscle running along the colon long axis.

The tarsal bone with which the tibia and fibula articulate to produce the ankle joint. The talus is also the key of the medial longitudinal arch of the foot.

The strong medial (deltoid) collateral lig of the ankle joint has tibionavicular, tibiocalcaneal and tibiotalar components. The deltoid lig is so strong that the medial malleolus of the tibia may break before the ligament.

Literally, the support of the talus, a shelf of bone projecting from the medial side of the calcaneum.

Anatomical Names	Latin/Greek or Other Origins	Examples
		Talocalcaneo-navicular joint
Tarsus, tarsal, tarso-	**Tarsos**: [Gr] *flat of the foot, instep*	Tarsal bones
		Tarsometatarsal joints
Tectorial	**Tectorium**: [L] *a covering*	Tectorial membrane
Tectum	**Tectum**: [L] *roof, ceiling, cover*	Tectum
Tegmen, tegmentum	**Tegmen[tum]**: [L] *covering, shelter, roof*	Tegmentum
		Tegmen tympani
Temporal, temporalis, temporo-	**Tempora**: [L] *the temples of the head*	Temporal bones
		Temporal lobe
		Temporal or temporalis m
		Temporomandibular joint
Tension, tensor	**Tendere**: [L] *to stretch, spread, strain*	Tensor (fascia lata, tympani, veli palatini) mm

Notes, Links and Non-Anatomical Usages

This is a multi-axial compound joint allowing gliding and rotational movements. Inversion and eversion of the foot involve this joint.

Tarsus, metatarsus, metatarsal. The 7 bones of the tarsus (what are their names?) form the ankle and bony arches of the foot. Tarsiers are insectivorous Primates with very long tarsal bones.

These are roughly plane synovial joints between the metatarsal bones and the distal (cuneiform and cuboid) tarsal bones.

The tectorial membrane of the vertebral column is a continuation of the posterior longitudinal lig and inserts on the occipital bone. It forms a roof over the dens of the atlas. Another tectorial membrane is made of gelatinous material and forms a covering over the hair cells of the organ of Corti of the inner ear.

Detective (someone who uncovers things!). The tectum or roof of the midbrain bears the corpora quadrigemina.

Integument, tegument. The tegmen[tum] of the midbrain is separated from the crus cerebri by substantia nigra. Together, these 3 components make the cerebral peduncle.

The tegmen tympani is a thin plate of temporal bone which forms a roof for the mastoid antrum, tympanic cavity and canal of the tensor tympani m.

Temporal bones underlie the temporal region.

The temporal lobes lie in the middle cranial fossa. With what special senses are they associated and what is their arterial supply?

The muscle arises from the bone of the temporal fossa and its fibres converge to descend deep to the zygomatic arch to insert on the coronoid process of the mandible. The muscle is supplied by the mandibular division of cranial V n. What are its actions?

This is a bicondylar ellipsoid joint between the temporal articular tubercle and anterior part of the mandibular fossa (above) and mandibular condyle (below). An articular disc divides the joint into upper and lower parts. The complex allows elevation, depression, protrusion, retraction and side-to-side (chewing) movements. What muscles produce these actions?

Tension, tensile, tensor (all these muscles stretch things, i.e. the fascia lata of the thigh, the tympanic membrane or the soft palate respectively). A tendon takes the strain!

Anatomical Names	Latin/Greek or Other Origins	Examples
Tentorium	**Tentorium**: [L] *tent*	Tentorium cerebelli
Teres	**Teres**: [L] *long and round, cylindrical*	Teres minor m
		Pronator teres m
		Ligamentum teres
Tertius	**Tertius**: [L] *third*	Peroneus tertius m
Thalamus, thalamic	**Thalamus**: [L] *inner room, bedroom*	Thalamus
		Interthalamic adhesion
Thenar, hypothenar	**Thena**: [Gr] *palm of the hand*	[Hypo]thenar mm [Hypo]thenar eminence
Thyroid, thyro-	**Thyreos**: [Gr] *oblong shield*; **eidos**: [Gr] *shape*	Thyroid cartilage
		Thyrocervical trunk
		Thyroidea ima a
Tibia, tibial[is], tibio-	**Tibia**: [L] *shinbone, flute*	Tibia

Tent. The tentorium cerebelli is a sheet of dura mater overlying the cerebellum in the posterior cranial fossa.

Teres muscles tend to be rounded or cylinder-like. Teres minor and major mm produces movements at the shoulder joint. Which ones?

The pronator teres is a relatively long cylinder arising by humeral and ulnar heads between which runs the median n. The muscle attaches to the midshaft of the radius on its lateral side. Are there any other pronators to assist it?

The free edge of the falciform lig contains the round lig which, before birth, was the left umbilical v. After birth, it becomes a fibrous cord called the ligamentum teres or round lig of the liver. Other round ligaments are associated with the ovary and uterus. What do they represent?

Tertiary. There are 3 peroneal mm in each set and this is the third in importance. Peroneus tertius m is anatomically more related to the extensor digitorum longus m and is a dorsiflexor of the foot.

The thalamus is a major inner region of grey matter in the cerebrum and a relay station but not for olfaction.

Joins the left and right thalamus.

The thenar eminence actually forms the fleshy part of the palm of the hand at the base or ball of the thumb. The thenar mm are found within this eminence. The hypothenar eminence is the less prominent (hypo- indicates below) medial or ulnar fleshy ridge running from wrist to little finger. The hypothenar mm underlie this eminence.

Thyroxine. The thyroid cartilages 'shield' the larynx anteriorly.

This arterial trunk arises from which part (1st, 2nd or 3rd) of the subclavian a? Its branches (inferior thyroid, transverse cervical and suprascapular aa) supply the inferior part of the thyroid gland, structures in the neck and muscles on the dorsal surface of the scapula.

Ima: [L] lowest. Hence, the lowest of the arteries supplying the thyroid gland. The others are?

The medial long bone of the leg, forming the shin.

Anatomical Names	Latin/Greek or Other Origins	Examples
		Tibial n
		Tibialis posterior m
		Tibiofibular joints
Trabecula, trabeculae, trabecular	**Trabecula**: [L] *little beam, strut*	Trabeculae carneae
		Trabecular bone
Trachea, tracheal, trachealis	**Trachos**: [Gr] *rough*	Trachea
		Tracheal cartilages
		Trachealis m
Trapezius, trapezium, trapezoid	**Trapezion**: [Gr] *table*; **eidos**: [Gr] *shape*	Trapezius m

This is one of the 2 main divisions of the sciatic n. It pursues a straight course on the posterior aspect of the leg, first on fascia covering the tibialis posterior m and then on the tibia itself. At the distal end of the tibia, it runs deep to the flexor retinaculum and behind the medial malleolus to divide into the medial and lateral plantar nn of the foot.

The deepest of the deep muscles of the posterior compartment of the leg. It arises from the interosseous membrane and adjacent bones and passes behind the medial malleolus of the tibia to insert where in the foot? Remember, it is the main invertor, and a powerful plantar flexor, of the foot.

The proximal joint (between the lateral condyle of the tibia and head of the fibula) is almost plane. The distal joint is a syndesmosis. What ligaments are associated with these bones and joints?

Trabeculae carneae are muscular roughenings of the ventricular walls of the heart and are covered in endocardium. They are better developed in the left ventricle. They appear as irregular ridges, columns, bands or protrusions.

In contrast to compact bone, sections of trabecular bone show spaces criss-crossed by bars or struts whose patterns are related to the lines of stress to which the bones are exposed.

Actually an abbreviation of trachea arteria (rough artery) so somebody was fooled into thinking it was an artery but had noticed it was rougher than normal (due, clearly, to the many C-shaped rings of cartilage!). Trachoma (inflammation and a graininess of the conjunctiva). At what level does the trachea bifurcate into the main bronchi?

The trachea is kept patent by C-shaped rings of cartilage which are deficient posteriorly. The lowest cartilage has an inferior ridge (the carina) which runs downwards and backwards between the left and right main bronchi. The isthmus of the thyroid gland joins the 2 lobes and crosses the second and third tracheal cartilages.

A transverse band of smooth muscle which runs between the posterior ends of tracheal cartilages and lies between the trachea and oesophagus.

A trapezium is a quadrilateral with one pair of sides or with no sides parallel. The latter more closely describes the shape of the muscle. Trapeze (usually quadrilateral).

Anatomical Names	Latin/Greek or Other Origins	Examples
		Trapezium
		Trapezoid
Triceps	**Triceps**: [L] *three-headed*	Triceps brachii m
Tricuspid	**Tricuspid**: [L] *having three points*	Tricuspid valve
Trigeminal	**Trigeminus**: [L] *threefold, triple, triplet*	Trigeminal n
Trigone	**Trigonus**: [L] *triangular*	Trigone
Triquetral	**Triquetrus**: [L] *three-cornered, triangular*	Triquetral bone
Trochanter, trochanteric	**Trekhein**: [Gr] *to run, roll*; **trokhos**: [Gr] *wheel*	Greater and lesser trochanters
		Intertrochanteric crest
Trochlea, trochlear	**Trochlea**: [L] *pulley*	Trochlea of the humerus
		Trochlear n (cranial IV)
Tuber, tubercle, tuberosity	**Tuber**: [L] *lump, swelling, protuberance*	Omental tuber
		Infraglenoid tubercle

Notes, Links and Non-Anatomical Usages

A carpal bone distinguishable by its shape. It has a tubercle to which the flexor retinaculum attaches (so the retinaculum goes from the hook of the hamate to the tubercle of the trapezium!).

A bone between the capitate and trapezium bones of the wrist.

The 3 heads of the triceps m are long, medial and lateral and their fibres run together to form a tendon which inserts on the olecranon. What are the origins of the 3 heads?

The valve has 3 cusps which form the atrioventricular valve on the right side of the heart. How do the papillary mm and chordae tendineae help this valve to close during systole?

Cranial V n. The triplet of trigeminal branches: the ophthalmic, maxillary and mandibular divisions.

Trigonal, trigonometry. The trigone of the bladder is a smooth triangular area with the internal urethral and 2 ureteric orifices at its angles.

A triangular carpal bone on the distal palmar surface of which sits the pisiform bone.

The term trochanter was originally applied to the rounded head of the femur which rotates, like a wheel, in the acetabulum. Nowadays, it refers to the two bony processes of the proximal end of the femur. What muscles and ligaments attach to the greater and lesser trochanters?

The bony ridge on the posterior aspect of the femur which runs between the 2 trochanters. The quadrate tubercle lies on this crest.

The trochlea of the distal end of the humerus is shaped like a pulley and articulates with a notch on the ulna.

The trochlear n supplies the superior oblique m of the eyeball. This muscle has its line of pull altered by a small fibrous loop, the trochlea, on the frontal bone at the superomedial angle of the orbit.

Tuber, protuberance, tubercular, tuberosity. The omental tuber is on the inferior or visceral surface of the liver to the right of the gastric impression and to the left of the caudate lobe. The slight prominence is so-called because it is in contact with the lesser omentum.

A lump related to the inferior part of the rim of the glenoid fossa of the scapula. To it is attached the long head of triceps brachii m. It is worth noting that the long head of biceps brachii m runs to a comparable supraglenoid tubercle!

Glossary 2   **113**

Anatomical Names	Latin/Greek or Other Origins	Examples
		Deltoid tuberosity
Tunica	**Tunic**: [L] *coat*	Tunica vaginalis testis
Tympanic, tympano-	**Tympanum**: [L] *drum, tambourine*	Tympanic membrane
		Epitympanic recess
		Tympanosquamous fissure

U.

Anatomical Names	Latin/Greek or Other Origins	Examples
Ulna, ulnar, ulnaris	**Ulna**: [L] *elbow, arm*	Ulna
		Ulnar n
		Flexor carpi ulnaris m
Umbilicus, umbilical	**Umbo**: [L] *boss of a shield*; **umbilicus**: [L] *little boss or navel*	Umbilicus
		Paraumbilical vv
Uncus, uncinate	**Uncus**: [L] *hook, crooked, curved*	Uncus

Notes, Links and Non-Anatomical Usages

A roughened area of bone on the middle of the lateral aspect of the humeral shaft into which the tendon of the deltoid m inserts.

Tunicate (marine animal with a body surrounded by a jelly-like coat). The tunica vaginalis of the testis is a serous sac invaginated by the testis and lying deep to the 3 layers of spermatic fascia. Its visceral and parietal layers are continuous posteriorly.

Tympani (set of kettledrums). The tympanic membrane is often called the eardrum.

The epitympanic (above the eardrum) recess is the part of the tympanic cavity lying above the tympanic membrane.

Sometimes called the squamotympanic fissure, this narrow fissure separates the superior tympanic part of the temporal bone from the posterior part of the articular portion of the mandibular fossa.

The ulna is actually the medial long bone of the forearm and not of the arm.

Arises from the medial cord of the brachial plexus and supplies muscles in the forearm and hand and skin on the medial (ulnar) side of the hand and medial 2 fingers.

One of only 2 muscles in the forearm which are innervated by the ulnar n. This muscle is a flexor of the wrist and lies on the medial (ulnar) side of the wrist. The pisiform bone develops as a sesamoid bone in its tendinous insertion.

Umbilicus (the little boss of the belly, 'belly-button'), umbilical. What spinal level is represented by the dermatome which includes the umbilicus? An alternative way of dividing the abdomen is to describe 4 quadrants via a vertical and a horizontal line, each of which passes through the umbilicus. The plane corresponding to the horizontal line (the transumbilical plane) passes through the disc between vertebrae L3 and L4.

Passing 'alongside the umbilicus', these veins connect veins of the anterior abdominal wall with those of the left portal v extending along the ligamentum teres in the falciform lig. It is these paraumbilical vv which distend to form the caput Medusae in portal hypertension.

The uncus is a hook-like part of the hippocampal gyrus.

Anatomical Names	Latin/Greek or Other Origins	Examples
		Uncinate process
Ureter, ureteric	**Ourein**: [Gr] *to urinate*	Ureter
		Ureteric constrictions
Urethra, urethral	**Ourein**: [Gr] *to urinate*	Urethra
		Urethral sphincter m
Uro-	**Oura**: [Gr] *urine*; **ourein**: [Gr] *to urinate*	Urogenital triangle
		Urothelium (urinary or transitional epithelium)
Utricle, utriculus	**Utriculus**: [L] *little bag*	Prostatic utricle
		Utriculus of the inner ear
Uvula, uvulae, uvular	**Uva**: [L] *grape*; **uvula**: [L] *little grape*	Uvula (palate, cerebellum)
V.		
Vagina, vaginal[is]	**Vagina**: [L] *sheath, scabbard*	Vagina
		Vaginal a

The hook-shaped part of the pancreatic head that lies posterior to the origin of the superior mesenteric vessels and arises from the ventral pancreas.

The ureters pass urine from kidney to bladder.

Constrictions found typically at 3 sites. Where are they?

The urethra passes urine from bladder to outside the body.

This sphincter is voluntary (after early infancy!) and controls the passage of urine.

Urine, urinal, urinary, urinate, etc. Generally, uro- implies related to the urinary system. The urogenital triangle is the anterior region of the perineum, the posterior being the anal triangle. The anterior triangle is defined by lines joining the pubic symphysis and 2 ischial tuberosities.

Transitional epithelium is stratified but the apparent number of layers varies according to the degree of stretch or distension.

The prostatic utricle opens on an elevation called the colliculus seminalis on the posterior wall of the male urethra. Embryologically, the utricle corresponds to the uterus and vagina.

The utricle or utriculus of the inner ear is the larger of 2 sacs (the other being the saccule or sacculus) lying in the vestibule of the membranous labyrinth.

The uvula of the soft palate is a median conical process which hangs inferiorly from the posterior border. It may be elevated and retracted by a bilateral muscle (the musculus uvulae) which is supplied by the pharyngeal plexus. The uvula of the cerebellum is part of the inferior cerebellar surface between the pyramid and nodule.

A sheath or scabbard accommodates the blade of a knife, sword, etc. No prizes for guessing what the anatomical 'blade' might be!

This is a branch of the internal iliac a. It descends in front of the ureter to the base of the broad lig and, at the lateral vaginal fornix, crosses superior to the ureter. It supplies branches to the vagina, cervix, uterus and uterine tubes.

Anatomical Names	Latin/Greek or Other Origins	Examples
		Pubovaginalis m
Vagus, vagal	**Vagus**: [L] *wandering, rambling*	Vagus n (cranial X)
		Vagal nuclei
		Vagal trunks
Vallecula, valleculae	**Vallis**: [L] *valley*	Vallecula epiglottica
Varicose, varicosity	**Varicosus**: [L] *full of swollen veins*	Varicose vv
Vas, vasa, vaso-	**Vas**: [L] *vessel, vase*	Vas deferens
		Vasa vasorum
		Vasodilation
Vastus	**Vastus**: [L] *monstrous, great, desolate, waste*	Vastus medialis m
Vein, vena, venae, venous	**Vena**: [L] *vein, blood vessel, way*	Internal jugular v

Notes, Links and Non-Anatomical Usages

This muscle constitutes part of the levator ani m in females and acts as a vaginal sphincter muscle. The pubic part of levator ani is divisible into 3 sets of fibres that run downwards, posteriorly and medially. The medial part is pubovaginalis m. What are the other parts called?

Vagabond (no fixed abode), vagary (erratic idea or action), vagrant (a wanderer), vague (not fixed, absent-minded). The vagus n is so-called because of its extensive wandering course innervating structures between the cranium and midgut.

The vagus n has 4 nuclei in the medulla oblongata: the dorsal nucleus (visceral efferent, parasympathetic), nucleus ambiguus (somatic efferent), nucleus solitarius (visceral afferent) and spinal trigeminal nucleus (somatic afferent).

The anterior vagal trunk is formed mainly from the left vagus n and enters the abdomen on the anterior surface of the oesophagus and sends branches to the stomach, pylorus and liver. The right vagal trunk is formed mainly from the right vagus n on the posterior of the oesophagus. Branches supply the stomach, coeliac and superior mesenteric plexuses, and intestines as far as the splenic (left colic) flexure.

Vallecula (literally, little valley). The vallecula epiglottica on each side forms a valley between the median and lateral glossoepiglottic folds. These mucosal folds run between the tongue and epiglottis.

So...it's the legs, not the veins, that are varicose!

Vase, vasomotor, vasopressin. The vas deferens runs between the epididymis and common ejaculatory duct via the superficial inguinal ring, inguinal canal and deep inguinal ring.

Vasa vasorum (vessels of the vessels).

Dilation of a blood vessel. This and vasoconstriction are brought about by vasomotor fibres innervating smooth muscle in the vessel wall.

Vast, devastation. The vastus medialis m arises from the intertrochanteric line and linea aspera of the femur. It inserts into the quadriceps tendon and patella. It is supplied by the femoral n. What are its actions?

Vein, venous, venesection. The internal jugular v begins at the jugular foramen as a continuation of the sigmoid sinus. It descends in the carotid sheath (which contains what other important structures?) and ends by joining the subclavian v to form a brachiocephalic v.

Anatomical Names	Latin/Greek or Other Origins	Examples
		Portal venous system
		Venae cavae
Ventral	**Venter**: [L] *belly, stomach, protuberance*	Ventral
Ventricle, ventricular	**Ventriculus**: [L] *small belly, stomach*	Ventricle
		Atrioventricular node
Vermiform	**Vermis**: [L] *worm*	Vermiform appendix
Vertebra, vertebrae, vertebral	**Vertebra**: [L] *a joint, especially of the backbone*	Vertebra
		Vertebral aa
Vesicle, vesicular, vesical, vesico-	**Vesica**: [L] *bladder, ball*	Seminal vesicle
		Vesical plexus
		Vesico-uterine pouch
Vestibule, vestibulo-	**Vestibulum**: [L] *porch, entry, vestibule*	Vestibule (inner ear, larynx, nose)
		Vestibulocochlear n (cranial VIII)

The tributaries of the portal v are the splenic, inferior mesenteric, superior mesenteric, gastric (left and right) and cystic vv.

Both the SVC and IVC enter the right atrium of the heart. What areas do they drain?

Ventriloquist. Ventral and anterior are often used interchangeably.

The cerebral and cardiac ventricles are obvious examples but they are not so-named because they are stomach-shaped.

The node is found in the lower part of the interatrial septum just above the attachment of the septal cusp of the right atrioventricular valve of the heart.

Vermicelli (looks, but doesn't taste, like worms!), vermiform, vermifuge (a drug which kills intestinal worms), Vermouth comes from the shrub wormwood (absinth, a potent green alcoholic drink also had a high wormwood content but was banned because of toxic effects. It is now becoming fashionable again!). The vermiform appendix is aptly named.

Ultimately, from vertere: [L] to turn. The vertebral joints also allow flexion and extension movements. Aversion, version, vertigo.

Arise from which part of the subclavian aa? Each vertebral a runs through the foramina transversaria of cervical vertebrae (except C7) and enters the skull via the foramen magnum. What artery is formed when the 2 vertebral aa unite?

Each seminal vesicle develops from the ampulla of the vas deferens with which it forms the ejaculatory duct. The vesicles can be palpated anteriorly via the anal canal.

Pelvic autonomic nn distributed to the bladder.

In females, peritoneum is reflected from the anterior of the uterus to the superior surface of the bladder to create a shallow pouch.

The vestibules of the inner ear, larynx and nasal cavities are merely entrances to those spaces.

Leaves the middle cranial fossa via the internal auditory (acoustic) meatus to supply organs of hearing (audition) and balance (equilibration).

Anatomical Names	Latin/Greek or Other Origins	Examples
Vinculum, vincula	**Vinculum**: [L] *bond, tie*; **vincula**: [L] *chains*	Vinculum
Viscus, viscera, visceral	**Viscus**: [L] *internal organ, intestines, bowels, inmost part*	Viscus
		Visceral pericardium
Vitreous	**Vitreus**: [L] *glassy*	Vitreous body
Vomer	**Vomer**: [L] *ploughshare*	Vomer
Vulva	**Vulva**: [L] *wrapper, womb*	Vulva

X.

Xiphisternum or xiphoid process	**Xiphos**: [Gr] *sword*; **eidos**: [Gr] *shape*	Xiphisternum Xiphoid process

Z.

Zygoma, zygomatic	**Zygos**: [Gr] *yoke*	Zygoma, zygomatic bone

Notes, Links and Non-Anatomical Usages

Vincula are found at various sites but all are 'connective' tissues such as those which attach flexor digitorum tendons to the phalanges.

Eviscerate (disembowel). Visceral and splanchnic both refer to the organs of the body.

Serous membranes usually have visceral (covering the organ) and parietal (lining the walls) components separated by a fluid-filled sac. Visceral pericardium covers the heart and corresponds to epicardium.

Vitrify (to turn to glass). Vitreous humour is found in the vitreous body which accounts for about 80% of eyeball volume. It forms a colourless, transparent gel of somewhat glassy appearance.

The vomer is a ploughshare-like bone forming the postero-inferior part of the nasal septum.

Vulvitis. Vulva is a collective term, like pudenda, used to describe the mons pubis, labia, clitoris, vestibule and vestibular glands of the female genitalia. So it actually excludes the womb!

The 2 names are interchangeable. The manubrium (handle), body (blade) and xiphoid process (tip) together resemble a short sword favoured by the Roman and Greek soldiers.

2 names used to identify the bones which give the prominences to the cheeks and form the inferolateral margins of the orbits. They are joined to which other bones of the skull? The reason for their likeness to a yoke is a mystery to me still!

INDEX FOR GLOSSARY